MALNUTRITION
Its causation and control

MALNUTRITION
Its causation and control
(with special reference to protein calorie malnutrition)

Volume 2

John R. K. Robson
School of Public Health
University of Michigan

in collaboration with

Frances A. Larkin
Anita M. Sandretto
Bahram Tadayyon

GORDON AND BREACH

NEW YORK   LONDON   PARIS

John R. K. Robson, M.D. (Newcastle), D.T.M. & H. (Edinburgh), D.P.H. (London), is Professor of Human Nutrition, and Director of the Nutrition Program, at the School of Public Health, The University of Michigan, U.S.A.;

Frances A. Larkin, Ph.D. (Cornell), M.S. (Minnesota), is Associate Professor of Nutrition, at the School of Public Health, The University of Michigan, U.S.A.;

Anita M. Sandretto, M.P.H. (Michigan), is Instructor in Nutrition at the School of Public Health, The University of Michigan, U.S.A.; and

Bahram Tadayyon, Ph.D. (Cornell), M.S. (American University of Beirut), is Associate Professor of Biochemistry, Faculty of Sciences, at Mashad University, Mashad, Iran.

To Benjamin Stanley Platt (1903–1969)
Professor of Human Nutrition

Contents

Preface

We have been involved in various aspects of nutrition work in every continent of the world. This experience, which covers a range of eighteen years, has included the planning of nutrition programs at national and local levels and the delivery of nutrition services in the richest and the poorest countries of the world. Our experience has covered laboratory and field research, and teaching nutrition in a variety of settings from graduate and undergraduate programs in nutrition in the United States and elsewhere, to the training of local auxiliaries in the field.

It is our impression that a vast amount of information has been accumulated but there is less evidence of application through the establishment of effective nutrition programs. We believe that an understanding of the environment is a prerequisite for the application of knowledge to nutrition problems regardless of whether the site is in Africa, Asia, or in an "inner city ghetto" in the United States. We perceive that one of the greatest needs is a better understanding of the interrelationships of the various factors which influence nutritional status. Knowledge of nutritional science will not be used effectively unless it is related to physiology, pathology, human behavior, and the many factors constituting the ecology of food and nutrition. Our combined experiences have led us to believe that there is a need for a textbook that will examine some basic principles in nutrition as related to the environment. The causation and control of malnutrition differs little in principle between the developing and sophisticated areas of the world. The latter situation is more complex and therefore it is more difficult to isolate and identify all the factors related to causation and control. In an attempt to recognize the breadth of the problem, we have therefore addressed ourselves to discussing several questions. What are the manifestations of malnutrition, what is the setting? What is normal nutrition and what nutrients does the body require to maintain health? How do we know if adequate nutrition has been achieved? How do we promote better nutrition and relieve existing malnutrition? These questions are discussed separately in each chapter. A systematic approach to the study of each disease has been avoided, as we believe such an approach tends to inhibit an understanding of the interrelationships. We make no apologies for the fact that the reader has to consult separate sections of the book in order to obtain a complete understanding of one specific problem such as the causation and control of protein calorie malnutrition.

It seems apparent to us that a broad concept of nutrition is required but we hope that we have made it clear that breadth does not necessarily mean that depth of understanding has to be sacrificed. Our attitudes, views, and understanding of nutrition have been acquired through an exposure to a number of scholarly and human personalities in nutrition and we would like to acknowledge their role in stimulating the writing of this book. In addition to the late Professor B. S. Platt to whom this book has been dedicated, we would like to express our particular appreciation to Dr. George Wadsworth, Professor Emeritus, University of Singapore, and A. G. van Veen, Professor Emeritus, Cornell University who have provided us with guidance, counsel, and an understanding of human nutrition. We would also like to acknowledge the help of colleagues scattered throughout the world including Professor H. A. P. C. Oomen, Dr. David Morley, Dr. J. M. Tanner, Mrs. Joyce Doughty of the London School of Hygiene and Tropical Medicine, Dr. J. M. Bengoa of the World Health Organization and Dr. Marcel Autret and Dr. Bruce Nicholl of the Food and Agriculture Organization who have provided photographs or figures. Finally we would like to thank Simon Robson for his help with art work, and our respective wives, husbands, and relatives for their support. We also wish to express our appreciation to our indefatigable secretary Mrs. Gertrude Flint, our associate Mrs. Elodia Jones, Cleland Child and Tom Raboine who always helped when help was most needed.

J. R. K. R.

CHAPTER 4

Nutrient requirements

Normal nutrition is dependent on the body being supplied with essential nutrients in the correct amount and proportions at the time the nutrient is required. The amounts and proportions are dependent on numerous inherited, environmental, and physiological influences described in previous sections.

The term requirement is used very loosely, consequently it may have several meanings. In its first usage, it refers to the *absolute requirement* of the body for a particular nutrient. The amount may depend on the weight, size, age, sex, physiological or pathological status of the individual. The amount is related to individual characteristics, and it may be impossible to determine with any degree of accuracy the quantity of this *absolute requirement*. For example a man aged 30 years weighing 70 kg with a calorie expenditure of 3,000 calories may have an *absolute requirement* for thiamine of 0.60 mg per day. If his weight increases or his calorie expenditure rises, then his *absolute requirement* will also increase.

The body may have problems in meeting this *absolute requirement* because of other extraneous factors. For example the *absolute requirement* for thiamine depends on the proportion of calories being provided by carbohydrate and fat. If the diet is predominantly carbohydrate the metabolic machinery will require extra thiamine. There is, therefore, a new requirement for thiamine that is related to existing circumstances. The *absolute requirement remains the same*, the *conditioned requirement is greater*. Similarly the *absolute requirement* for vitamin A may be 0.4 mg. If however, 0.4 mg of vitamin A are given in a fat-free diet, the *absolute requirement* for the body will not be met because only a small part of the vitamin A will be absorbed. The *absolute requirement* for vitamin A remains at 0.4 mg but because of the present circumstances a *conditioned requirement* has now been established. To insure the *absolute requirement* is met, the *conditioned requirement* may have to be many times greater. Because it is difficult to ascertain the *absolute requirements* it is virtually impossible to make accurate predictions for the needs for any one nutrient on an individual basis.

There is no doubt however, that nutritionists require rules and guide-lines for evaluating nutrient intakes, and planning diets; as the following discussion will show, nutrient requirements are frequently arbitrarily defined.

Definitions

A nutrient requirement is the quantity of a particular nutrient the body must have in order to function properly. Since the required amount of a nutrient varies from one individual to another, and varies in one individual under different conditions, quantitative estimates of requirements should always be related to these conditions. This means the requirement should be expressed in relation to age, sex, nutritional status, size, and physiological state. It should also be quite clear whether the requirement is being expressed at minimal or optimal levels.

Minimum requirement

This is the *least* amount of an ingested nutrient that will prevent symptoms or clinical signs of nutrient deficiency, maintain biochemical levels in tissues and tissue fluids commensurate with a normal healthy state, and will also maintain normal physiological function.

The clinical symptoms and signs are illustrated by the lesions of scurvy that are characteristic of vitamin C deficiency, and bone abnormalities associated with rickets in vitamin D deficiency. It is questioned whether prevention of clinical deficiency symptoms and maintenance of "normal" biochemical responses actually measure the same state of nutrition. Is the minimum requirement of a nutrient the smallest amount that will prevent deficiency disease? Or, is it an amount that will support function when there has been cellular adaptation of the cells, tissues, and organs to a diminishing nutrient supply? To maintain normal cell function in nutrient depletion, there must be adaptation of the metabolic processes. However, when the adaptation becomes permanent this may represent an abnormal function. The true minimum requirement for nutrients probably lies somewhere between an initial shift to alternative metabolic pathways and the final sign of failure to adapt, usually shown as clinical disease. At the present time a true minimum requirement for the various nutrients cannot be precisely defined.[1]

Average requirement

When a group of individuals is considered, the requirements for any one nutrient for each member of that group will cover a range of values. The average of these values may be taken as an average requirement. The actual requirement of an individual in the group may be above, below, or the same as that requirement.

The terms minimum· requirement and average requirement are often used indiscriminately, resulting in some confusion. Quite clearly, however, the former relates to adequacy in individuals and the latter, to adequacy in groups.

Estimates for minimum and average requirements have been based on data obtained from a limited number of subjects who may not be truly representative of the population. This raises some doubt about the propriety of their extrapolation to large numbers of people or population groups.

Optimum requirement

The optimum requirement is the amount of a nutrient which will assure an individual the best possible health, functional capacity and resistance to disease. In order to evaluate such a requirement quantitatively, all the physiological functions of each nutrient would have to be measured, and scientists would have to know the function(s) most susceptible to deficiency, or the function that has priority over others. Unfortunately, the science of nutrition has neither identified, nor rated in order of importance, all the functions of nutrients.[2]

Minimum daily requirements

The minimum requirement as defined, should not be confused with the *Minimum Daily Requirements*, that appear on the commercial wrappers of foodstuffs in the United States. The *Minimum Daily Requirements* are legal standards, established by the Federal Food and Drug Administration for labelling foods and pharmaceutical preparations that have special dietary uses. These standards specify the amounts of certain nutrients, especially vitamins, which are considered necessary for the prevention of deficiency diseases. The *Minimum Daily Requirements* were first stated in the Federal Register on November 22, 1941, and have been supplemented by addenda published periodically since that time. However, they are applied to only a limited number of vitamins and minerals (see Table 30). The original regulations specify how the quantities of nutrients, especially vitamins, are to be expressed on food labels. The vitamins are measured in United States Pharmacopia units, commonly referred to as U. S. P. units. One U. S. P. unit equals one International Unit (I. U.), a measure that is used more commonly in other parts of the world.

1*

Table 30 Minimum daily requirements of specific nutrients

Nutrient	Infants	Children 1–6 years	Children 6–12 years	Adults 12 and over	Pregnancy or lactation
Vitamin A (USP)	1500	3000	3000	4000	
Thiamine, mg	0.25	0.50	0.75	1.00	
Riboflavin, mg	0.60	0.90	0.90	1.20	
Niacin, mg		5	7.5	10	
Ascorbic acid, mg	10	20	20	30	
Vitamin D (USP)	400	400	400	400	
Calcium, gd		0.75	0.75	0.75	1.50
Phosphorus, g		0.75	0.75	0.75	1.50
Iron, mg		7.5	10	10	15
Iodine, mg		0.1	0.1	0.1	0.1

Source: U. S. Food and Drug Administration.

Dietary allowances

Nutrient requirements refer to individuals but because there is no simple method of assessment, it is not practical to determine the nutrient requirements for each person in a population. Because of individual variation, as well as uncertainty about the nutrient needs for optimum health, an increment (safety factor) is usually added to the average nutrient requirement. The value represented by the requirement plus the safety factor is known as a *Recommended Dietary Allowance* (RDA); it should be adequate for individuals in population groups with needs greater than average.[3]

Many countries have adopted *Dietary Standards*. These are numerical expressions of the quantities of the various nutrients considered necessary to maintain adequate health and nutrition in the various age and physiological groups of the population.

The first attempt to define nutritional requirements on an international basis was made under the leadership of the League of Nations. After the demise of the League of Nations at the outbreak of the second World War, the specialized agencies of the United Nations assumed responsibility for advising on this subject. The World Health Organization has prepared *recommended daily intakes* for vitamins A and D, thiamine, riboflavin, niacin, ascorbic acid, vitamin B_{12}, folate, and iron (see Table 31). These are analogous to the *recommended dietary allowances* of national governments.

National dietary allowances or *Dietary standards* are used in making food policies and plans to insure that the majority of the people have diets

Table 31 Recommended daily intakes of vitamins and iron

Nutrient	Recommended intake per day	Comment
Vitamin A	750 µg retinol	1 I. U. of Vitamin A = 0.3 µg retinol
Thiamine	0.40 mg per 1000 Calories	
Riboflavin	0.55 mg per 1000 Calories	
Niacin	6.6 niacin equivalents per 1000 Calories	60 mgs of tryptophan= 1 mg niacin
Ascorbic acid		
Birth–12 years	20 mgs	
13 years and over	30 mgs	
Pregnant women	50 mgs	
Lactating women	50 mgs	
Vitamin D		
Birth–6 years	10 µg	2.5 µg of cholecalciferol
7 years and over	2.5 µg	= 100 I. U. of vitamin D
Pregnancy	10 µg	
Lactation	10 µg	
Vitamin B$_{12}$		
Birth–12 months	0.3 µg	
1–3 years	0.9 µg	
4–9 years	1.5 µg	
10 years and over	2.0 µg	
Pregnancy	3.0 µg	
Lactation	2.5 µg	
Folate		
Birth–6 months	40 µg	
7–12 months	60 µg	
1–12 years	100 µg	
13 and over	200 µg	
Pregnancy	400 µg	
Lactation	300 µg	
Iron		
Birth–4 months	0.5 mg	
5–12 months	1.0 mg	
1–12 years	1.0 mg	
13–16 years (boys)	1.8 mg	
(girls)	2.4 mg	
Women	2.8 mg	
Men	0.9 mg	
Pregnancy	2.8–6.6 mg	Depends on state of iron depletion

Source: W. H. O. Tech. Rep. Series Nos. 362 and 452.

that will maintain health. The recommendations depend on the criteria used to define dietary adequacy, the interpretation of the published work dealing with human nutritional requirements, the estimates of biological variation within the population, and the effects of stresses in normal everyday living. *Dietary standards* are intended for people having dietary habits and dietary practices typical of that country and living under the same environmental conditions. Any dietary allowances or recommended intakes intended for international use must be modified in accordance with the physical and demographic characteristics of the country. Not unnaturally, there are differences between national and international recommendations, but these-differences are gradually being reduced as more knowledge accumulates and the dietary allowances are revised.[4]

Recommended Dietary Allowances have been developed for the United States and are under continuing review by the National Research Council through the Food and Nutrition Board. The objective of the allowances has been to provide a guide, or standard, for the maintenance of good nutrition of healthy persons of all ages and both sexes living under "normal" conditions in the United States. The *Recommended Dietary Allowances* have been effective for the purposes of planning the diets of groups or institutions and for determining food policies of enrichment or supplementation. Other countries have a different safety factor built into their recommended dietary standards.

Experimental methods designed to determine nutrient requirements of humans

Several kinds of studies can be used for determining human nutrient requirements, including balance studies, biochemical measurements of nutrients or nutrient metabolite levels in tissues and tissue fluids, and clinical evaluations and performance tests.

Balance studies

Principles The principle of conservation of energy and matter serves as a basis for metabolic studies since they compare the nutrient intake and output (or loss) from the body. Only stable nutrients or nutrients with easily recognizable metabolic end products are suitable for use in this type of study. Data have been obtained from energy, mineral and protein (nitrogen) balance studies. Vitamins are not suitable for this type of study since a great variety of metabolic end products may be formed. The human body can also synthesize some vitamins and their availability may seriously interfere with the interpretation of results.

The balance method can be simplified to the following equation:

$$Balance = Intake - Excretion\ Products.$$

Excretion products are those substances lost by way of the intestinal tract and kidney or through the lungs and skin.

The data obtained from balance studies are expressed as positive balance, negative balance, or equilibrium. A positive balance is a condition of bodily gain of a nutrient; a state of net gain occurs when the ingestion of a nutrient is greater than its excretion. A negative balance is the opposite condition; the body is excreting more of the nutrient or its metabolic products than is being ingested. In these circumstances, the level of ingestion is assumed to be too low to replace nutrient losses from the body, or to prevent the withdrawal of nutrients from the body tissues.

Withdrawing nutrients from body tissues in an effort to make up nutrient deficiencies may provide temporary relief, but tissue damage may result. Equilibrium is representative of a steady state when ingestion and excretion of nutrients are, for all practical purposes, equal. All these terms refer to the overall economy of the body and give no indication of exchanges between, and within, individual cells.

Limitations of balance studies   Two problems must be taken into account when conducting balance studies. These are the effect of previous intake and adaptation. Balance studies are very much influenced by the previous levels of intake of a nutrient. Individuals who are accustomed to diets providing ample protein will go into negative balance at a much higher level of intake than others who have been consuming smaller amounts of protein. Adaptation presents much the same type of problem since humans can adapt to varying levels of nutrient intake. Calcium intake, for example, varies widely in different parts of the world but persons may be in equilibrium regardless of high or low dietary intakes, the latter group having adapted to a lower level of intake. The amount of adaptation that can take place varies according to the nutrient involved. The interval of time for adaptation also varies; it may occur within days for some nutrients[5], but adaptation to changes in calcium intake may require several months.[6]

The ability to adapt means that changes can take place during metabolic studies which may invalidate the results.

Special problems in determining vitamin requirements

The determination of vitamin requirements presents special problems. Because of their variety, no single method of assessing requirements gives satisfactory results for every vitamin. Several different methods of investigation are used to determine vitamin requirements, including nutrition surveys which usually include a clinical evaluation. The methods also include biochemical tests that measure enzyme activity, or the levels of vitamins or vitamin metabolites, in the tissues fluids. In some tests, the urinary excretion, or blood level, may be measured following a test dose of the vitamin to be studied.

Not only are different tests used for different vitamins, but there are probably several different stages of vitamin nutriture. The stages may be summarized as follows:

Tissue saturation
↓
Tissue de-saturation
↓
Biochemical deficiency signs
↓
Clinical Deficiency signs

The above sequence of events may take place when a healthy, well nourished person is placed on a diet deficient in a single vitamin and is then observed during well controlled experimental deprivation.

Ideally, measurement of nutrients should be made at every level up to, and including, the stage of clinical deficiency; however, in most experimental conditions there may be technological problems that prevent this. Very sensitive tests are available for some vitamins but not others. Because of differences in the metabolic function of vitamins, some measurements may have to be made on blood levels and others on urinary metabolites. The type of measurement, and its feasibility in all stages of deprivation, also depends on the available technology for measuring minute quantities of vitamins or vitamin metabolites.

The presence of these problems means that estimates for requirements for any one vitamin may be based on very different criteria and experimental procedures from those used to estimate requirements of other vitamins.

The measurement of the human requirement for a vitamin actually gives some indication of the body stores of that vitamin. Tissue saturation implies that an increase in the dietary intake of a vitamin will not increase the tissue stores of the vitamin significantly. Thus a state of "optimal" nutrition is implied. This concept is useful in relation to the water soluble vitamins, but has little meaning when applied to the fat soluble vitamins. The nature of the body pool or tissue stores differs for each vitamin. The fat soluble vitamins are stored primarily in the liver, whereas the bulk of the water soluble vitamins appear in the muscle mass. The blood vitamin content may, or may not, be in equilibrium with the other body stores. Similarly the urinary excretion of a vitamin is not a valid measure of requirements when the metabolic state is changing rapidly.[7] The term vitamin requirement can be defined either as the amount of the vitamin necessary to prevent deficiency disease, or the amount necessary to maintain a certain level of the vitamin, or its metabolites, in the blood or urine. These requirements may obviously not be numerically the same. For this reason, when any requirement is stated, the methods used for evaluation of the requirement should be stated.

Biochemical measurements of nutrient or metabolite levels

Principles The principle goal in biochemical tests is to achieve measurements that reflect the total metabolic pool. The levels of the various nutrients should be a true reflection of the nutritional status of the organism.

In laboratory animals, but not humans, certain organs can be removed and analyzed for nutrients or metabolites. In humans, other tissues and tissue fluids may be analyzed, the substrate depending on the nutrient. In order that the data may be correctly interpreted, the origins of the substrate should be identified, for one site may provide more representative data than another for a particular nutrient. For example, the liver, which is the reserve pool for 90 per cent of vitamin A, reflects vitamin A status more accurately than blood. Conversely, blood gives a better assessment of thiamine levels than liver.[8] Usually the substrate that is most readily available is used; in humans this may include blood, urine, feces, liver, skin, and adipose tissue.

Limitations of biochemical methods Blood specimens can be collected with relative ease as they contain nutrients which may be moving throughout the body and into, and out of, cells. However, the presence of nutrients in the blood is not always indicative of nutritional status; nutrient levels are subject to change, depending on recent intakes of food and the presence of other nutrients. For example, calcium levels in the blood are dependent on phosphate cations; when the phosphate cations are diminished serum calcium anions increase.

Urine specimens are more difficult to collect; they contain nutrients and metabolites. Theoretically, there should be a good correlation between excretion of nutrients and nutrient intake. The higher the intake, then the greater should be the excretion of the nutrient, and this is certainly true of some of the water soluble vitamins. Thiamine, for example, is linearly related to the intake except at low levels.[9] There is individual variability however, and it has been observed that the excretion varies among groups of individuals having the same intake.

With vitamin C, the urinary excretion approximates the intake when the body is saturated with the vitamin (i.e. when the tissue stores can no longer be increased[10]).

The excretory products of protein and minerals provide a good index of intake but, with vitamins, it is almost impossible to equate intake with catabolic products. Thiamine is excreted in several forms with only a small part being excreted as free thiamine.[7] Some vitamins when broken down may be excreted by the feces as well as the urine.

Although laboratory conditions can be standardized and controlled, physiological responses cannot; consequently, fluctuations in levels of nutrients and metabolites in tissue fluids may occur during balance studies. When this happens, the validity of the data must be affected.

Clinical evaluation

Principles   Clinical evaluation of humans (a subject discussed in the next chapter) can be used to detect and diagnose lesions caused by nutritional deficiences. A clinical evaluation is particularly useful for studies of vitamin requirements. The clinical course of vitamin deficiency can be studied also in subjects who are carefully maintained on controlled levels of vitamin intake. Such studies, conducted over a period of months, can provide estimates of the amount of a particular vitamin necessary to prevent frank deficiencies. In order to give a more complete picture of the nutritional status of the total human organism, the data from clinical evaluations should be correlated with biochemical analyses from blood and urine.

Limitations   The greatest problem associated with clinical evaluation is the subjective judgement of the individual examiner. Examiners may not agree on the criteria for the recognition, and interpretation, of signs of nutrient deficiencies. Unless criteria are standardized, error will be inevitable.

Performance tests

Fitness tests, which include observations on endurance, reflex action, and psychological response, have been used to measure body function. Fitness tests may detect physical changes before frank deficiency symptoms appear and they have been used to determine thiamine requirements.

Psychological tests have also been used to detect changes during nutrient deprivation, but the reaction of the subject may be due as much to the testing regime as to changes in the nutrient intake.

Choosing the appropriate test

Sometimes the actual function of the vitamin is unknown; this makes experimental determination of requirements difficult. The physiological functions of pyridoxine for example, are not fully understood, so it is difficult to know experimentally whether deprived subjects are suffering from dysfunction or not. Ascorbic acid, on the other hand, has so many functions that it may be difficult to decide which function should be tested and whether the test provides the most appropriate index of ascorbic acid status.

The determination of ascorbic acid requirements relies primarily on biochemical assessment of the degree of tissue saturation.

When humans have a known constant intake, equilibrium occurs between the intake and body stores. At high levels of intake (75–100 mg per day) there is an increase in the plasma concentration of ascorbic acid. The white blood cell-platelet concentration of ascorbic acid, which reflects the degree of tissue saturation, seems to reach a maximum at a level of 30 mg of ascorbic acid per 100 mg of white cells. When tissue saturation is approached, the urinary excretion of the vitamin is approximately the same as the intake.

During loading tests, the plasma concentration is measured before, and at regular intervals after, a test dose of vitamin is given. Loading tests are done to show how much vitamin C is required to bring the biochemically deficient state up to a state of saturation.

In all these tests, unless the intake of ascorbic acid has been constant, the plasma level probably reflects the variations in recent intake more than the degree of body or tissue saturation.

Despite the amount of knowledge that has accumulated on vitamin C levels in the blood, and other tissues, the question of human requirements for ascorbic acid remains unanswered. Is the requirement the amount of the vitamin that will produce a certain plasma or white blood cell-platelet concentration, or is it the amount which will produce tissue saturation?

The recommendations for the dietary intake of ascorbic acid range from 30–75 mg per day, depending on the age of the person and, in the case of females, whether they are pregnant or lactating. There is evidence however, that ascorbic acid intake of 10–15 mg per day will prevent scurvy.[11]

Because of the known variations in human needs, the recommended intake of the vitamin is greater than the intakes that will prevent scurvy.

Energy requirements

The energy necessary for human survival is obtained from food in the form of calories. The need for energy varies from person to person. Each individual has a total caloric requirement that includes the energy needed to maintain body processes, physical activity, the energy of specific dynamic action and the energy needed to maintain body temperature.

Because each person is different, the total caloric intake must be adjusted to the specific needs of the individual. In adults, the total caloric requirement is being met when the caloric intake maintains body weight. In children, the requirements are satisfied when the rate of growth is maintained at desirable levels over an extended period of time. Allowances are intended to provide the *absolute calorie* needs of healthy individuals, and they do not take into account additional stress associated with injury, infection, or disease. When these are present, the *conditioned calorie* need is increased to provide energy for tissue repair, for immunological mechanisms, and to compensate for the wasting effects of fever.

Energy needed to maintain body processes

The energy needed to maintain body processes includes the energy to maintain basal metabolism and the synthesis of new tissue in growth or repair.

The numerous factors that affect the Basal Metabolic Rate have been described in the previous chapter (see page 243). The additional energy needs for growth are considerable; they are constantly changing (see Table 32).

Table 32   Changes in proportion of total energy expenditure on growth

	Infancy			Childhood	
	At birth	3 months	1 year	2 years	9–11 years
Percentage total energy spent on growth	40	40	20	20	4–10
Average weight (kgs)	3	5	10.4	12.4	27.1
Average height (cms)	50	58	73	84	129

Source: McNaught, A. B. *Companion to Illustrated Physiology*, p. 35. Williams and Wilkins, Baltimore, 1965.

Energy for physical activity

Physical activity involves muscular work. This is the most variable factor in the energy requirements of individuals. In a moderately active person, physical work probably represents about one-quarter of the total energy expenditure. In a very active person, the energy needed for muscular work could exceed the energy needed for the basal metabolism. The amount of energy used in physical activity is proportional to the work done. This in turn depends on the type of activity, the size of the individual, the amount of time spent on the activity, and the efficiency with which the task is performed. Relatively small amounts of energy are required for such activities as sitting, writing, studying, or driving a car. Much larger amounts of energy are required for walking, riding a bicycle, swimming, or other active sports. To the dismay of students, it has been established that mental effort demands no extra energy.

In developing countries where energy sources may be in short supply, considerable amounts of energy may be expended in daily household tasks and in work that might not be a necessary part of life in the highly industrialized societies.

The grinding of grain, the collection of firewood and carrying water (and a child) sometimes a distance of several miles requires the expenditure of considerable quantities of energy. In addition to this there are tasks in the field that involve hard work (see Table 33). The demand for energy is subject to seasonal variations depending on the state of the crop. The monthly variation in energy expenditure in the Gambia is shown in Table 34.

The size of a person creates a definite variation in the amount of energy needed for an activity. More energy is required to move a large body. Training is important as greater efficiency in the work operation can be achieved by practice. The training may involve economy of required move-

Table 33 Energy expenditure for individual operations during the production of rice

Operation	Energy expenditure Cals/hr/kg body weight
Hoeing and broadcasting seed	3.2
Weeding	2.4
Thinning seedlings	2.1
Scaring birds	1.0
Harvesting	1.7

Source: Fox, R. H. Ph. D. Thesis, London University.

Table 34 Energy expenditure of Gambian farmers

Estimated energy expenditure per head per day by month of the year

Month	BMR SDA*	Other activities	Crop cultivation	Total energy expended
2	1245	300	0	1575
3	1245	150	0	1395
4	1245	150	0	1395
5	1245	150	210	1605
6	1245	150	512	1907
7	1245	150	540	1935
8	1238	150	363	1751
9	1238	150	291	1679
10	1231	150	279	1660
11	1231	150	79	1460
12	1238	300	220	1760
1	1238	300	173	1711

* SDA = Specific Dynamic Action
Source: Fox, R. H., Ph. D. Thesis, London University.

ment or economy of non-purposive movement and may result in considerable conservation of energy.

The energy of Specific Dynamic Action (SDA)

This has been discussed in the previous chapter. It is the increase in heat
production after the ingestion of food. The amount of heat produced
depends on the quantity and quality of the food, the basal metabolic rate
of the subject, and the nutritional state of the individual.

It has been noted that convalescent malnourished infants produce more
heat after meals than infants who have completely recovered from malnutrition.[12] This not only indicates that the Specific Dynamic Action may
be associated with two kinds of heat production but there is also an extra
requirement for SDA in early recovery from protein calorie malnutrition.

Energy needs for adjustment to the environment

There is evidence that the energy cost of work increases by about five
per cent in ambient temperatures below about 57°F. In addition there is
a two to five per cent increase in energy expenditure associated with carrying
the extra weight of cold-weather clothing and footgear. Such clothing
also slightly increases energy expenditure by its "hobbling" effect. If the

body is inadequately clothed, body-cooling will occur, and calorie needs will increase because of the increased voluntary movement. In addition, there is a tendency to increase activity in cold climates and to decrease activity in hot weather.

Energy requirements are increased also during work at high temperatures (about 99 degrees F). Under such conditions the body temperature and the metabolic rate increases and the body expends extra energy in its efforts to maintain thermal balance. Little adjustment appears to be necessary for change in moderate environmental temperature between 68–86 degrees F.

Estimating calorie requirements

Several techniques have been used to estimate calorie requirements; these are based on the consumption of calories in food, or the expenditure of energy.

The computation of calorie intake from the dietary intake can be inaccurate for several reasons. First, it is difficult to make an accurate estimate of food consumption. Even if good data can be obtained, the computation of calories may be fallacious because not all of the food may be utilized by the body. Many of the computations are based on the calorific value of the food as determined by bomb calorimetry; this value represents the total caloric value of the food and includes indigestible materials, such as fiber, that make no contribution to the calorie utilization.

Daily energy expenditures are calculated from the summation of energy used in all the different types of activity throughout the day. Although the energy expenditure of a given activity can be determined with a high degree of accuracy in an individual (see page 242), the amount of energy expended on a particular activity varies from person to person. It is difficult, furthermore, to make accurate estimations of time spent on specific activities and it may also be difficult to categorize some of them. Because of these problems, a scale of recommended allowances, based either on food consumption or energy expenditure, must contain some degree of inaccuracy.

Alternative scales have been suggested using a theoretical, healthy, human, living in a temperate climate as a basic standard.[13]

The *Reference Man* weighs 65 kg, is 25 years of age, free of disease and physically fit for active work, and he lives in a temperate climate having a mean annual temperature of 10 degrees Centigrade. He is in calorie balance and works 8 hours a day; during this time he is involved in hard labor only occasionally. He is sedentary for 4 hours and may walk for up to 1–1/2 hours and he spends a similar amount of time on recreation. He is assumed to require, on average, 3,200 calories daily throughout the year. The *Reference Woman* is similar, her weight is 55 kg and she is also

25 years of age, engaged in light physical activity, walks for one hour and engaged in recreation for 1 hour. She requires on average, 2,300 calories per day throughout the year.

For an individual the total energy requirement based on body size can be calculated from the formula

$$E = 152 \, W^{0.73} \text{ for men and}$$

$$E = 123.4 \, W^{0.73} \text{ for women,}$$

where E = total energy requirement and W = nude weight in kg. Having determined the total calorie requirement, adjustments can be made for age and environmental temperature.

Similar calculations can be used to determine the requirements of infants, children and adolescents. Calorie requirements can be expressed as total calories per unit of body weight (see Fig. 82).

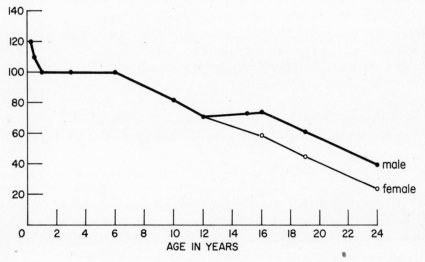

Figure 82   Calorie requirement by age and body weight (Data from FAO Nutritional Studies, No. **15**, 1957). Vertical axis shows kilocalories per unit body weight.

The total calorie requirement increases with age; it reaches a maximum during puberty, decreases thereafter until maturity, and reaches a plateau during adult life (see Figure 83). In females this may be interrupted by pregnancy and lactation. During pregnancy, extra energy is needed for the growth of the fetal and maternal tissues, as well as for moving the increased body mass. The need for extra energy may be met by ingesting more food, by reducing physical activity, or by doing both.

An increased intake of 200 Calories per day for pregnant women has been recommended.[14] During lactation, extra energy is needed for the production of milk. The efficiency of human milk production has been estimated at 60 per cent. In order to supply sufficient calories in breast milk, it was usual for mothers to be encouraged to consume an additional 1000 Calories per day during lactation. Recent work suggests that the efficiency of milk production in humans is as high as 90 per cent;[15] if this is correct an extra 600 Calories per day would meet the needs of lactation. Aging is accompanied by a reduction in the total calorie requirement.

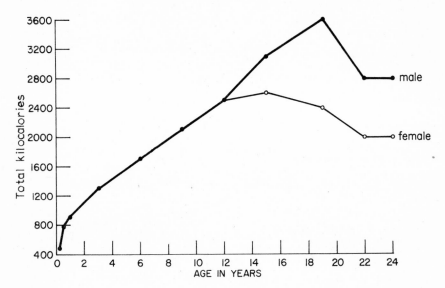

Figure 83   Calorie requirement by age (Data from FAO Nutritional Studies, No. **15,** 1957)

The assessment of calorie requirement in an individual is obviously liable to subjective decisions relating to activity. When attempts are made to assess the energy requirements of whole populations the difficulties are magnified.

The population has to be divided into groups according to age, sex, physiological status, and activity. The respective needs for each of the groups may be calculated and then added together; adjustments may then be made for climate and environment. Inevitably errors enter into computations on calorie requirements, and it is important that the nutritionist avoids making a diagnosis of caloric undernutrition when comparing the calorie intake of individuals or small groups with the recommended allowances for whole populations.

Requirements for individual nutrients

Absolute requirements and recommended dietary allowances

Absolute requirements and recommended dietary allowances are tabulated at the end of this chapter. The definition and specification of minimum requirements and dietary allowances are far more complicated than a casual perusal of the recommendations might suggest. It is important for the nutritionist to understand the problems that face research workers, in their efforts to define requirements. For some nutrients, the accurate estimation of requirements is almost impossible. In well-intentioned attempts to define a minimum level of intake, the figure that has been arrived at may already include a safety factor whose magnitude is unknown. Nevertheless, an additional safety factor is added, so the allowance for some nutrients may be quite unrealistic. The terms *minimum requirement* and *dietary allowance* are used quite loosely in many publications and the student should be aware of the duplicity of interpretation of these terms.

Some of the units of measure are extremely small; this tends to introduce a false sense of accuracy into some of the recommendations. It should be remembered that several of the levels of intake have been decided quite arbitrarily, and they may be far removed from the absolute level. Many of the recommendations have been based on the results of research that is difficult to conduct and control. Several major procedural and technical difficulties have to be overcome during experimentation. There are also many problems in interpreting the data because of the interrelationship of nutrients. While research workers continue to provide data to establish adequate levels of intake, populations continue to live in good health on levels of intakes below those determined experimentally as minimum levels.

In the following discussion the determination of minimum requirements and dietary allowances for some individual nutrients will be used to illustrate some of the problems.

Protein requirements

Human protein requirements are influenced by age, body size, quality of the protein, the caloric content of the diet and special physiological needs.

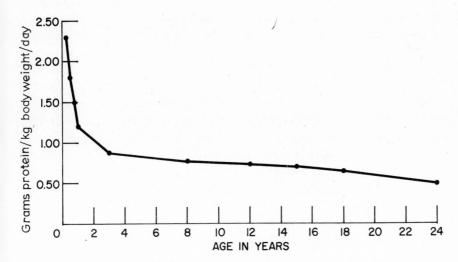

Figure 84   Reference protein requirements by age (Data from World Health Organization Technical Report Series No. **301,** 1965)

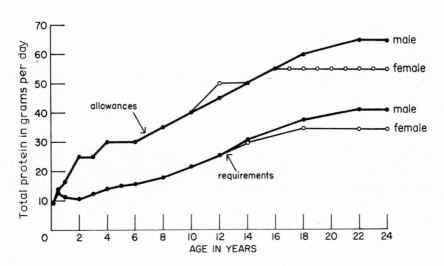

Figure 85   Protein requirements and recommended dietary allowances by age and sex (Data from World Health Organization Technical Report Series, No. **301,** 1965 and *Recommended Dietary Allowances*, Seventh Edition, National Academy of Sciences, Washington D. C. 1968)

Age   The influence of age is especially evident in early life when protein is needed for building new tissues during growth. The protein requirement of infants and young children is considerable when expressed per unit of weight. However, the total amount of protein needed by the smaller body of the infant or child is much less than the total amount needed by an adult. As the age of the child increases and he enters a period of less rapid growth, the protein needs are less per unit of body weight than they are during infancy. This trend continues through childhood but there is a subsequent rise during adolescence. A plateau is reached in adult life and maintained until old age when there may be an increase in demands (see Figure 84).

The need expressed as total grams of protein has a reverse trend. During fetal life and infancy the total need is small, but it increases with age until adult life (see Figure 85).

The protein requirement therefore reflects changes in the rate of growth during the life cycle and additional physiological demands.

Physiological demands   The protein needs of the pregnant or lactating mother are obviously greater than those of other adult women. During pregnancy she must ingest sufficient protein to provide for her own needs as well as for the needs of the growing fetus. During lactation, she must also supply the protein used in the synthesis of milk.

Body size   An increase in body size increases the need for protein, especially during adolescence and early adult life. The total amount of protein needed for tissue repair and maintenance is dependent on the amount of active tissue in the body, especially muscle tissue. The protein need is expressed per unit of body weight and the amount required per unit body weight is the same for both sexes. Since the male is usually larger and heavier than the female, he will need more *total* protein.

Muscular work   Once the body has been trained, and muscle developed for the task, hard physical work seems to have no appreciable effect on the protein requirement. There is no scientific justification for providing extra protein for the man who is doing muscular or hard physical work other than that needed to meet the cost of obligatory losses and incidental trauma.

Quality and quantity of protein in the diet   Protein serves as a source of amino acids for building tissues during growth and for maintaining and repairing tissues during adult life. Protein can also provide energy when other nutrient sources (fats and carbohydrates) are inadequate. The human body does not require protein *per se* but it requires specific amounts and proportions of the essential amino acids contained in proteins. Accordingly, it is necessary to define the requirements of the human for amino acids. A deficit in protein quality can never be made up by providing extra amounts of the same protein for an imbalance of essential amino acids will persist. Deficiencies in quality of one protein can only be compensated by providing other proteins that supply the deficient amino acids. When only protein of low biological value is available, it is usually present in the food in low concentrations. Because of this, practical difficulties arise in consuming enough of the food to meet the quantitative needs for protein. When cassava, banana, or yam provide the basis of the diet, satiety may be reached before the protein requirements can be met.

Through various experiments, the approximate needs for the essential amino acids of various age groups have been determined. This original research was followed by further investigation of the amino acid content of food sources of proteins. The only natural foods identified as having an ideal amino acid pattern meeting human requirements, are human milk, and whole eggs. In comparison to these, other food sources of proteins have been ranked according to their amino acid content.

Proteins are classed as having a high, or low biologic value according to their ability to supply the essential amino acids required by the human body (see page 215).

Special needs Both malnutrition and illness can cause depletion of protein from body tissue, and extra protein is needed by a person recovering from illness.

Estimating protein requirements

Protein requirements are usually determined by one of three methods; the first ascertains the amount of an essential amino acid required to maintain nitrogen balance in subjects receiving an otherwise adequate diet. The second establishes the amount of protein required to maintain nitrogen balance at varying levels of intake, and the third estimates the obligatory losses of nitrogen from the body.[16]

There are limitations to each of these methods. For example, when there is a deficiency of an essential amino acid, new tissues cannot be synthesized since all the essential amino acids must be present at one time for protein biosynthesis to proceed. The bulk of the protein and amino acids in the diet are therefore metabolized and excreted in the urine. The body, when depleted of an exogenous source of an essential amino acid, utilizes its own tissues. However, the other amino acids, freed at the same time in the process of tissue catabolism, are available in excess so they are degraded and excreted. In states of depletion, the extent of the negative nitrogen balance is greater therefore than the actual loss caused by the deficiency of one essential amino acid.

There may be priorities with in the metabolic machine so a shortage of one of the nine essential amino acids may cause a greater amount of tissue wastage than others. Further studies are required on this subject before the protein requirements can be accurately estimated from essential amino acid deprivation studies.[17]

In nitrogen balance studies, the protein intake may be varied and the nitrogen excretion measured against the level of the dietary protein intake. By these means, the amount of protein required to maintain nitrogen balance is interpreted as the protein requirement of that person. However, the body can adapt to a lowered protein intake. Although there may be a temporary period of negative nitrogen balance, equilibrium may be restored at this lower level of intake.

If the intake is reduced again, the body will once more go into negative nitrogen balance and further adaptation may take place. It follows that compensatory adaptation should be completed before the protein requirement is determined experimentally. The ability of the body to adapt appears dependent on the levels of protein intake prior to the deprivation. Persons on a high intake go into negative nitrogen balance on a higher level of intake than subjects who have habitually consumed a low protein intake.

The experimental data may also be affected by the use of synthetic or semi-synthetic diets that are not normally consumed during life.

The amino acids and proteins contained in diets are released during digestion. The physical and chemical nature of the protein, other nutrients present in the digestive tract, and the digestive process itself, may affect the release of amino acids. In any one situation, neither the quantity nor quality of the amino acids available to the body is known.[18] In these circumstances it may be appreciated that it is no easy task to estimate requirements accurately. It is possible that equally accurate predictions for requirements may be obtained by the *Factorial Method*. This depends on estimating *obligatory nitrogen losses* or the unavoidable losses of nitrogen from the body through the urine, feces, and skin. These losses occur during normal protein metabolism and turnover in the human body. Each loss is measured separately and then summated.

In addition to the obligatory nitrogen loss, an allowance is made (when necessary), for *stress*, and *new tissue formation* in *growing* children.

The general formula is $R = (U + F + S + G) \times 1.1$, where R = requirement, U = basal urinary loss, F = basal fecal loss, S = skin loss, and G = increment during growth. All the units are measured in mg of nitrogen per kg of body weight per day. The factor 1.1 represents an addition of 10 per cent to allow for stress. To obtain the protein equivalent of the nitrogen the value obtained is multiplied by the factor 6.25 (see page 214). Additional allowances can be made for the pregnant and lactating mother.

The protein requirements as specified by WHO and FAO and the Recommended Dietary Allowances of the National Academy of Sciences are compared in Figure 85. A more detailed comparison is shown in Table 35. The arbitrary nature of these recommendations may be seen when comparing the requirement and the recommended allowance for infants from birth to 2 months of age.

Table 35 Protein requirements and recommended allowances

Age group		Requirement* (grams/day)	Recommended allowance† (grams/day)
Infants:	0–2 months	Body wt (kg) × 2.3	kg × 2.2
	3–6 months	Body wt (kg) × 1.8	kg × 2.0
	6–9 months	Body wt (kg) × 1.5	kg × 1.8
	9–12 months	Body wt (kg) × 1.2	kg × 1.8
Children:	1–3 years	12	25
	4–6 years	15	30
	7–9 years	21	35
	10–12 years	26	45
Adolescents:			
Males:	13–15 years	34	50
	16–19 years	40	60
Females:	13–15 years	34	50
	16–19 years	36	55
Adults:			
Males:		38	65
Females		32	55
Pregnancy		+6	65
Lactation		+15	75

* *Protein requirements*. WHO Tech. Rep. Ser. No. 301, Rome, 1965.
† *Recommended dietary allowances*. 7th ed. Publication No. 1695, National Academy of Sciences. Washington, D. C., 1968.

Interrelationships of nutrients

The discussion on protein and calorie requirements illustrates how the nutrient needs vary from person to person and with the physiological changes occuring in different stages of the life cycle.

It is not proposed to make a systematic review of requirements for each nutrient. The reader seeking further information on requirements for specific nutrients is referred to standard texts on normal nutrition. In public health nutrition, it is the application of the knowledge pertaining to nutrient requirements that is of significance. In order that the most practical use may be made of nutrition knowledge, it is important to recognize how nutrient requirements are influenced not only by development and extraneous factors, but also by the presence, concentration, and function of other nutrients.

Interrelationships between nutrients will be summarized according to the type of interaction taking place.

Requirements determined by the availability of another nutrient

Interrelationships between the energy intake, protein intake, and several vitamins have been observed. In addition, there are also interactions between vitamins, between vitamins and minerals, and between vitamins and energy requirements that affect the respective requirements for these nutrients.

Thiamine The roles of thiamine, riboflavin, and niacin in energy metabolism are well recognized and documented; consequently, requirements of these vitamins are related to human energy needs and expenditures. There is evidence that not only is the requirement for thiamine related to the total calorie intake but also to the proportions of fat, carbohydrate, and protein in the diet. This is apparently due to the function of thiamine in the metabolism of carbohydrate. As the carbohydrate portion of the diet is increased, more thiamine is required for its metabolism. Conversely, thiamine requirements are reduced whenever other sources of calories are substituted for carbohydrates. For example, fat, protein, and alcohol have been reported to spare thiamine requirements.[19]

The total calorie requirement is related to body weight and age and the thiamine requirement varies accordingly. However, in old age thiamine needs be increased due to a decreased efficiency of utilization. Since energy expenditure increases in pregnancy, there is a greater need for thiamine. Additional thiamine may be utilized also in the metabolic process of milk production and secretion.

Riboflavin Riboflavin combines with protein in the body to form a labile compound that is one of a group of flavoproteins. The feeding of low protein diets under experimental conditions has been accompanied by an increased excretion of riboflavin and decreased tissue storage of that vitamin.[20] The association of riboflavin with protein in foods complicates balance studies of riboflavin requirements since foods that are inadequate in riboflavin are also likely to be deficient in protein.

When the body is in negative nitrogen balance or when protein metabolism is disordered, the limiting factor will probably be protein intake rather than riboflavin.

The results of animal experiments suggest that excess carbohydrate reduces the riboflavin requirements and an excess of fat increases the need for the vitamin. However, data are not available on humans.

It has been suggested that the riboflavin requirement is influenced by the oxygen consumption of the body and hence the energy turnover.[20]

Pyridoxine   Pyridoxine or vitamin B_6 is also involved in protein metabolism and the requirements for this vitamin are related to the protein intake. This is reflected in the increasing needs for pyridoxine in infancy through childhood into adult life and in pregnancy.

The presence of infections which initiate an antibody response creates extra demands for protein and therefore, pyridoxine.[21]

Vitamin A   The requirement for vitamin A is related to several other nutrients. The level of dietary fat is important as it facilitates the absorption of carotenes in the intestine. For example, fat represents less than 7 per cent of the total caloric intake in Ruanda in Central Africa. Although the diet there contains an ample supply of carotenes, these are inefficiently absorbed and vitamin A deficiency often appears. The addition of a small supplement of fat to the diet, markedly improves carotene absorption, increases serum vitamin A levels, and alleviates vitamin A deficiency.[22]

There are direct relationships between the level of protein intake and the need for vitamin A. It has been shown that utilization of vitamin A in the liver is directly proportional to the protein intake, when animals are fed a diet lacking vitamin A. It is suggested that dietary protein levels can affect vitamin A in two opposing ways. First, an ample allowance of protein will promote rapid growth which demands extra vitamin A. Second, a very low intake of protein can result in poor utilization of vitamin A since protein is necessary for its absorption, its mobilization in the liver, and its transport within the body. Vitamin A and carotenes are carried in the blood loosely bound to protein. It is possible therefore, that any condition which lowers serum protein levels might reduce serum vitamin A levels and produce a deficiency, despite adequate liver storage.[19] The interrelationship between protein and vitamin A is well exemplified in clinical practice since patients with kwashiorkor often have very low serum vitamin A levels. Provided there are adequate liver stores, the serum vitamin A rises in these cases on protein administration alone. This implies that the requirement for vitamin A can be dependent on the protein quantity and quality.

In areas where there is a high incidence of protein calorie malnutrition, treatment with a high quality protein may cause the resumption of growth and increase the vitamin A requirement. If the liver reserves of vitamin A are inadequate and if the intake of vitamin A or carotenes is not increased, vitamin A deficiency may become overt.

Where people live on a subsistence diet, limited primarily in protein and vitamin A, the development of vitamin A deficiency is slowed. This is due to a decrease in protein metabolism, decreased growth and a consequent reduction in vitamin A requirements.[23]

Other vitamins may affect the need for vitamin A. For example, vitamin E and ascorbic acid are natural antioxidants; they prevent randicity. In this role they help to avoid the destruction of vitamin A. If these vitamins are deficient, the need for vitamin A may be increased. Vitamin E may also be necessary for the absorption and utilization of vitamin A.[24]

Vitamin D   Vitamin D facilitates the absorption of calcium and phosphorus from the small intestine and aids in the normal deposition of these minerals in bones and teeth. Therefore, if the consumption of these minerals is increased, the need for vitamin D may be increased to aid in their utilization.

In addition to the need for fat to ensure the absorption of fat soluble vitamins, other nutrients in food may interact and increase the requirements of one, or the other, or both.

Ascorbic acid   Vitamin C facilitates the absorption of some of the iron in vegetables. Therefore communicies depending on vegetables as their source of iron may have a requirement depending on whether the ascorbic acid has been destroyed in cooking.

Calcium and phosphorus   The efficient use of calcium and phosphorus depends on the ratio of one mineral to the other. A calcium intake that is slightly greater than the phosphorus intake is optimal for utilization of both nutrients. A predominance of phosphorus is poorly tolerated and can lead to a loss of calcium, thereby increasing the requirements for this mineral.

Effect of dietary intake

Scientific study of requirements for some nutrients arrives at a minimum figure; sometimes it is higher than intakes known to maintain adequate health. Some of the reasons for this anomaly deserve further consideration. The discrepancy may be attributable to mistakes on computing intakes, or to technical problems in estimating the requirements, or perhaps both. The requirement for calcium, as determined by experimentation, is much higher than known intakes of calcium. For example, the requirements for growing children is estimated to be 75–150 mg per day. Experimental studies of the absorption of calcium limit the efficiency of absorption to a range of 15–35 per cent. In order to achieve an adequate intake at this range of efficiency, 500–800 mg of calcium should be ingested per day. It is known, however, that populations are living on intake levels as low as 250 mg per day in South Africa.[25] The ability of such populations to maintain adequate calcium status may be attributable to two factors. The first relates to the size of the skeleton; in many areas where diets are poor, the skeleton is small so the absolute requirement for calcium is less. Secondly, adaptation to low intakes of calcium takes place, and the efficiency of absorption and utilization of calcium is much greater. In addition to the physiological adjustments, in populations that are normally well fed there appears to be considerable individual variation in the ability to adapt. It is possible that in areas where calcium intakes are usually low, there may have been some genetic exclusion of individuals who could not adapt to low intakes.

The estimates of intake of calcium also present problems because phytates and oxalates in food may form insoluble compounds with calcium.

The estimated requirements for iron are influenced by the availability of iron in the food and also by the ability of the body to control iron absorption.

Despite low intakes of iron, an adequate status can be achieved by facilitated absorption of the element. This probably occurs during pregnancy or after blood loss. Estimates of iron requirements have been based on the status of iron stores and the measurement of iron losses in the feces, urine, skin, and sweat. As the studies have been mainly confined to adult males they give little insight into the requirements of infants and females. The former may have a deficient endowment at birth (see page 50). The latter have additional demands, caused by the loss of iron in the menses and in association with pregnancy and parturition.

Shared function of nutrients   The subject of protein calorie relationships has been discussed fully in Chapter 3. It can not be overemphasized that it is quite unrealisitic to assess protein adequacy on quantitative measurements. If there are inadequate calories in the diet, the deficit in energy sources will be made up from protein.

Niacin requirements are not only related to energy and protein intake, but also to amino acid intake, since the amino acid tryptophan can be converted in the body to niacin. Sixty mg of tryptophan are required for the synthesis of one mg of niacin. Tryptophan is a precursor of niacin, consequently the quality of the protein affects the niacin requirement. If good quality protein (a source of tryptophan) is available, the niacin requirement will be reduced because of the conversion of tryptophan to niacin. Some diets such as those based on maize are limited in biological value by the availability of tryptophan; there is, accordingly, an increased need for preformed niacin.

The requirement for vitamin A is affected by other nutrients in the food as well as those in the body. The dietary source of vitamin A affects the requirement because the vitamin can be obtained in either the preformed state, or as carotenes. The amount required to meet the need for the vitamin will depend on the form in which it is ingested. Because the body uses beta-carotene less eficiently than preformed vitamin A, a greater quantity of carotenes than preformed vitamin A must be ingested to meet the needs.

Biosynthesis of Vitamins

The requirement for vitamin K is unknown because of the ability of the micro-organisms of the intestinal tract to synthesize this vitamin. The newborn has no intestinal flora and is therefore unable to produce this vitamin. A single dose of one to two mg of vitamin K after birth will prevent deficiency.

Riboflavin, pyridoxine, and folic acid and vitamin B_{12} can all be synthesized by humans; however, the amount of the vitamin that is absorbed and utilized is not known.

Recommended intakes

The interrelationships of nutrients introduce variable factors that cannot be measured. Despite this, and the technical problems and difficulties in interpreting data, some guides are essential for the planning, monitoring, and evaluation of nutrition policies, programs and services. Tables 36, 37, and 38, show recommended daily allowances for nutrients in three countries. This has been prepared allowances for nutrients in three countries. This has been prepared from data from a variety of sources and accounts for the wide range of some nutrients.

Although these recommendations may not be a true reflection of nutrient needs, inaccuracies do not constitute a threat to human health provided

Table 36 Recommended daily nutrient intakes for Canadians

Sex	Age	Weight	Activity Category	Calories	Protein*	Calcium	Iron	Vitamin A	Vitamin D	Thiamine	Riboflavin	Niacin	Ascorbic acid
	yr.	lb.			gm.	gm.	mg.	I.U.†	I.U.	mg.	mg.	mg.	mg.
Both	0–1	7–20	usual	360–900	7–13	0.5	5	1,000	400	0.3	0.5	3	20
Both	1–2	20–26	usual	900–1,200	12–16	0.7	5	1,000	400	0.4	0.6	4	20
Both	2–3	31	usual	1,400	17	0.7	5	1,000	400	0.4	0.7	4	20
Both	4–6	40	usual	1,700	20	0.7	5	1,000	400	0.5	0.9	5	20
Both	7–9	57	usual	2,100	24	1.0	5	1,500	400	0.7	1.1	7	30
Both	10–12	77	usual	2,500	30	1.2	12	2,000	400	0.8	1.3	8	30
Boy	13–15	108	usual	3,100	40	1.2	12	2,700	400	0.9	1.6	9	30
Girl	13–15	108	usual	2,600	39	1.2	12	2,700	400	0.8	1.3	8	30
Boy	16–17	136	B‡	3,700	45	1.2	12	3,200	400	1.1	1.9	11	30
Girl	16–17	120	A§	2,400	41	1.2	12	3,200	400	0.7	1.2	7	30
Boy	18–19	144	B‡	3,800	47	0.9	6	3,200	400	1.1	1.9	11	30
Girls	18–19	124	A§	2,450	41	0.9	10	3,200	400	0.7	1.2	7	30
Male	adult	154	B	3,582	47	0.5	6	3,700	—	1.1	1.8	11	30
Female	adult	124	A	2,390	40	0.5	10	3,700	—	0.7	1.2	7	30

* Protein recommendation is based on normal mixed Canadian diet. Vegetarian diets may require a higher protein content.

† Vitamin A is based on the mixed Canadian diet supplying both vitamin A and carotene. As preformed vitamin A, the suggested intake would be about 2/3 of that indicated.

‡ Expenditure assessed as being 113% of that of a man of same weight and engaged in same degree of activity.

§ Expenditure assessed as being 104% of that of a woman of the same weight and engaged in the same degree of activity.

Source: Canadian Council on Nutrition.

Table 37 Food and Nutrition Board, National Academy of Sciences—National Research Council recommended daily dietary allowances*, (Revised 1968). Designed for the maintenance of good nutrition of practically all healthy people in the U. S. A.

	Age* (years) From Up to	Weight (kg)	Weight (lbs)	Height (cm)	Height (in.)	kcal	Protein (gm)	Vita-min A activity (IU)	Vita-min D (IU)	Ascor-bic acid (mg)	Fola-cin‡ (mg)	Nia-cin (mg equiv)§	Ribo-flavin (mg)	Thia-min (mg)	Vita-min B₆ (mg)	Vita-min B₁₂ (µg)	Cal-cium (g)	Iron (mg)
Infants	0–1/6	4	9	55	22	kg×120	kg×2.2††	1,500	400	35	0.05	5	0.4	0.2	0.2	1.0	0.4	6
	1/6–1/2	7	15	63	25	kg×110	kg×2.0††	1,500	400	35	0.05	7	0.5	0.4	0.3	1.5	0.5	10
	1/2–1	9	20	72	28	kg×100	kg×1.8††	1,500	400	35	0.1	8	0.6	0.5	0.4	2.0	0.6	15
Children	1–2	12	26	81	32	1,100	25	2,000	400	40	0.1	8	0.6	0.6	0.5	2.0	0.7	15
	2–3	14	31	91	36	1,250	25	2,000	400	40	0.2	8	0.7	0.6	0.6	2.5	0.8	15
	3–4	16	35	100	39	1,400	30	2,500	400	40	0.2	9	0.8	0.7	0.7	3	0.8	10
	4–6	19	42	110	43	1,600	30	2,500	400	40	0.2	11	0.9	0.8	0.9	4	0.8	10
	6–8	23	51	121	48	2,000	35	3,500	400	40	0.2	13	1.1	1.0	1.0	4	0.9	10
	8–10	28	62	131	52	2,200	40	3,500	400	40	0.3	15	1.2	1.1	1.2	5	1.0	10
Males	10–12	35	77	140	55	2,500	45	4,500	400	40	0.4	17	1.3	1.3	1.4	5	1.2	10
	12–14	43	95	151	59	2,700	50	5,000	400	45	0.4	18	1.4	1.4	1.6	5	1.4	18
	14–18	59	130	170	67	3,000	60	5,000	400	55	0.4	20	1.5	1.5	1.8	5	1.4	18
	18–22	67	147	175	69	2,800	60	5,000	400	60	0.4	18	1.6	1.4	2.0	5	0.8	10
	22–35	70	154	175	69	2,800	65	5,000	—	60	0.4	18	1.7	1.4	2.0	5	0.8	10
	35–55	70	154	173	68	2,600	65	5,000	—	60	0.4	17	1.7	1.3	2.0	5	0.8	10
	55–75+	70	154	171	67	2,400	65	5,000	—	60	0.4	14	1.7	1.2	2.0	6	0.8	10
Females	10–12	35	77	142	56	2,250	50	4,500	400	40	0.4	15	1.3	1.1	1.4	5	1.2	18
	12–14	44	97	154	61	2,300	50	5,000	400	45	0.4	15	1.4	1.2	1.6	5	1.3	18

14-16	52	114	157	62	2,400	55	5,000	400	50	0.4	16	1.4	1.2	1.8	5	1.3	18
16-18	54	119	160	63	2,300	55	5,000	400	50	0.4	15	1.5	1.2	2.0	5	1.3	18
18-22	58	128	163	64	2,000	55	5,000	400	55	0.4	13	1.5	1.0	2.0	5	0.8	18
22-35	58	128	163	64	2,000	55	5,000	—	55	0.4	13	1.5	1.0	2.0	5	0.8	18
35-55	58	128	160	63	1,850	55	5,000	—	55	0.4	13	1.5	1.0	2.0	5	0.8	18
55-75	58	128	157	62	1,700	55	5,000	—	55	0.4	13	1.5	1.0	2.0	6	0.8	10
Pregnancy					+200	65	6,000	400	60	0.8	15	1.8	+0.1	2.5	8	+0.4	18
Lactation					+1,000	75	8,000	400	60	0.5	20	2.0	+0.5	2.5	6	+0.5	18

* The allowance levels are intended to cover individual variations among most normal persons as they live in the United States under usual environmental stresses. The recommended allowances can be attained with a variety of common foods, providing other nutrients for which human requirements have been less well defined. See text for more-detailed discussion of allowances and of nutrients not tabulated.

† Entries on lines for age range 22–35 years represent the reference man and woman at age 22. All other entries represent allowances for the midpoint of the specified age range.

‡ The folacin allowances refer to dietary sources as determined by *Lactobacillus casei* assay. Pure forms of folacin may be effective in doses less than $1/4$ of the RDA.

§ Niacin equivalents include dietary sources of the vitamin itself plus 1 mg equivalent for each 60 mg of dietary tryptophan.

†† Assumes protein equivalent to human milk. For proteins not 100 per cent utilized factors should be increased proportionately.

Table 38 Recommended daily intakes of energy and nutrients for the United Kingdom

(a) Age range	Occupational category	(c) Body weight kg	(d) Energy kcal	(d) Energy MJ	(f) Protein g	(g) Thiamine mg	Riboflavine mg	(h) Nicotinic acid mg equivalents	Ascorbic acid mg	(i) Vitamin A µg retinol equivalents	(j) Vitamin D µg cholecalciferol	Calcium mg (l)	Iron mg (l)
Boys and Girls													
0 up to 1 year (b)		7.3	800	3.3	20	0.3	0.4	5	15	450	10	600	6
1 up to 2 years		11.4	1,200	5.0	30	0.5	0.6	7	20	300	10	500	7
2 up to 3 years		13.5	1,400	5.9	35	0.6	0.7	8	20	300	10	500	7
3 up to 5 years		16.5	1,600	6.7	40	0.6	0.8	9	20	300	10	500	8
5 up to 7 years		20.5	1,800	7.5	45	0.7	0.9	10	20	300	2.5	500	8
7 up to 9 years		25.1	2,100	8.8	53	0.8	1.0	11	20	400	2.5	500	10
Boys													
9 up to 12 years		31.9	2,500	10.5	63	1.0	1.2	14	25	575	2.5	700	13
12 up to 15 years		45.5	2,800	11.7	70	1.1	1.4	16	25	725	2.5	700	14
15 up to 18 years		61.0	3,000	12.6	75	1.2	1.7	19	30	750	2.5	600	15
Girls													
9 up to 12 years		33.0	2,300	9.6	58	0.9	1.2	13	25	575	2.5	700	13
12 up to 15 years		48.6	2,300	9.6	58	0.9	1.4	16	25	725	2.5	700	14
15 up to 18 years		56.1	2,300	9.6	58	0.9	1.4	16	30	750	2.5	600	15

Men												
18 up to 35 years	Sedentary	65	2,700	11.3	68	1.1	1.7	18	30	750	2.5	500	10
	Moderately active		3,000	12.6	75	1.2	1.7	18	30	750	2.5	500	10
	Very active		3,600	15.1	90	1.4	1.7	18	30	750	2.5	500	10
35 up to 65 years	Sedentary	65	2,600	10.9	65	1.0	1.7	18	30	750	2.5	500	10
	Moderately active		2,900	12.1	73	1.2	1.7	18	30	750	2.5	500	10
	Very active		3,600	15.1	90	1.4	1.7	18	30	750	2.5	500	10
65 up to 75 years }	Assuming a	63	2,350	9.8	59	0.9	1.7	18	30	750	2.5	500	10
75 and over }	sedentary life	63	2,100	8.8	53	0.8	1.7	18	30	750	2.5	500	10
Women												
18 up to 55 years	Most occupations	55	2,200	9.2	55	0.9	1.3	15	30	750	2.5	500	12
	Very active		2,500	10.5	63	1.0	1.3	15	30	750	2.5	500	12
55 up to 75 years }	Assuming a	53	2,050	8.6	51	0.8	1.3	15	30	750	2.5	500	10
75 and over }	sedentary life	53	1,900	8.0	48	0.7	1.3	15	30	750	2.5	500	10
Pregnancy, 2nd and 3rd trimester			2,400	10.0	60	1.0	1.6	18	60	750	10 (k)	1,200 (m)	15
Lactation			2,700	11.3	68	1.1	1.8	21	60	1,200	10	1,200	15

requirements and recommendations are recognized as estimates, and not incontrovertible. Recommended intakes in particular should never be used as a direct tool for evaluating nutritional status and it is unforgivable to assume that an individual or a group is malnourished because the intake of a nutrient does not appear to meet recommended levels. The assessment of nutritional status is a complex subject and will be discussed in the next chapter.

Footnotes to Table 38

(a) The ages are from one birthday to another: e.g. 9 up to 12 is from the 9th up to, but not including, the 12th birthday. The figures in the Table in general refer to the midpoint of the ranges, though those for the range 18 up to 35 refer to the age 25 years, and for the range 18 up to 55, to 35 years of age.

(b) Average figures relating to the first year of life. Energy and minimum protein requirements for the four trimesters are given in Tables 2 and 3 respectively.

(c) The body weights of children and adolescents are averages and relate to London in 1965. (Taken from Tanner, Whitehouse and Takaishi, 1966; Tables IV A and IV B, 50th centile.) The body weights of adults do not represent average values; they are those of the FAO (1957) reference man and woman, with a nominal reduction for the elderly.

(d) Average requirements relating to groups of individuals.

(e) Megajoules (10^6 joules). Calculated from the relation 1 kilocalorie = 4.186 kilojoules, and rounded to 1 decimal place.

(f) Recommended intakes calculated as providing 10 per cent of energy requirements (see paragraph 64). Minimum protein requirements given in Table 3.

(g) The figures, calculated from energy requirements and the recommended intake of thiamine of 0.4 mg/1000 kcal, relate to groups of individuals.

(h) 1 nicotinic acid equivalent = 1 mg available nicotinic acid or 60 mg tryptophan.

(i) 1 retinol equivalent = 1 μg retinol or 6 μg ß-carotene or 12 μg other biologically active carotenoids.

(j) No dietary source may be necessary for those adequately exposed to sunlight, but the requirement for the housebound may be greater than that recommended.

(k) For all three trimesters.

(l) These figures apply to infants who are not breast fed. Infants who are entirely breast fed receive smaller quantities; these are adequate since absorption from breast milk is higher.

(m) For the third trimester only.

Source: Reports on Public Health and Medical Subjects, No. 120. H. M. S. O., London, 1970.

References

1. Pike, R. L., Brown, M. *Nutrition an Integrated Approach*, p. 374. New York: Wiley 1967.
2. Couch, J. R., Davies, R. E. Vitamins B_1, B_2, B_6, Niacin and Ascorbic Acid. In *Newer Methods of Nutritional Biochemistry*, p. 215 Ed., Albanese, A. A. New York: Academic Press, 1963.
3. Hollingsworth, D. V. "Recommended Intakes of Nutrients for the United Kingdom." *J. Amer. Diet. Ass.* **56**: 200, 1970.
4. Patwardhan, V. N. "Dietary Allowances—An International Point of View." *J. Amer. Diet. Ass.* **56**: 191, 1970.
5. Allison, J. B. "Interpretation of Nitrogen Balance Data." *Fed. Proc.* **10**: 676, 1951.
6. Malm, O. J. "Calcium Requirements and Adaptation in Adult Men." *Scand. J. Clin. Lab. Invest.* (Supplement 36), **10**, 1958.
7. Pearson, W. N. "Blood and Urinary Vitamin Levels as Potential Indices of Body Stores." *Amer. J. Clin. Nutr.* **20**: 514, 1967.
8. Schaefer, A. E. "Symposium on Detection of Nutrition Deficiencies in Man." *Amer. J. Clin. Nutr.* **20**: 526, 1967.
9. Unglaub, W. G., Goldsmith, G. A. In *Methods for Evaluation of Nutritional Adequacy and Status*, p. 69. Spector, H., Peterson, M. S., Friedman, T. E. National Academy of Sciences, Washington, D. C. 1964.
10. Woodruff, C. W. Ascorbic Acid. In *Nutrition, A Comprehensive Treatise*, p. 288, Vol. **2**, Eds., Beaton, G. H., McHenry, E. W. New York: Academic Press, 1964.
11. Srikantia, S. G., Mohanram, M., Krishnaswamy, K. "Human Requirements of Ascorbic Acid." *Amer. J. Clin. Nutr.* **23**: 59, 1970.
12. Ashworth, A. "Malnutrition and Metabolic Rates." *Nutr. Rev.* **28**: 279, 1970.
13. Calorie Requirements, F. A. O. Nutritional Study No. 15, p. 10. F. A. O. Rome 1957.
14. *Recommended Dietary Allowances*. Seventh Edition, p. 7. National Academy of Sciences. Washington, D. C. 1968.
15. Thomson, A. M., Hytten, F. E., Billewicz, W. Z. "The Energy Cost of Human Lactation." *Brit. J. Nutr.* **24**: 565, 1970.
16. Brown, W. D. *Present Knowledge of Protein Nutrition*, p. 7. New York: Nutrition Foundation Inc. 1967.
17. Albanese, A. A., Orto, L. A. Proteins and Amino Acids. In *Newer Methods of Nutritional Biochemistry*, p. 7. Ed. Albanese, A. A. New York: Academic Press, 1963.
18. Wadsworth, G. R. Nutrition and Public Health. In *The Theory and Practice of Public Health*, p. 136. Ed. Hobson, W. Third Edition London: Oxford University Press, 1969.
19. Gershoff, S. N. "Effects of Dietary Levels of Macronutrients on Vitamin Requirements." *Fed. Proc.* **23**: 1077, 1964.
20. Bro-Rasmussen, F. "The Riboflavin Requirement of Animals and Man, and Associated Metabolic Relations." *Nutr. Abstr. and Rev.* **28**: 369, 1958.
21. Chow, B. F. The B Vitamins. In *Nutrition: A Comprehensive Treatise*, p. 207, Vol. **2**. Eds. Beaton, G. H., McHenry, E. W. New York: Academic Press, 1964.
22. Roels, O. A. *Present Knowledge of Vitamin A*, p. 51. New York: Nutrition Foundation, Inc., 1967.

23. Arroyave, G. "Inter-relations Between Protein and Vitamin A and Metabolism." *Amer. J. Clin. Nutr.* **22**: 1119, 1969.
24. Ames, S. R. "Factors Affecting Absorption, Transport, and Storage of Vitamin A." *Amer. J. Clin. Nutr.* **22**: 934, 1969.
25. Walker, A. R. P. "Nutritional, Biochemical, and Other Studies on South African Populations." *So. Afr. Med. J.* **40**: 826, 1966.

CHAPTER 5

The Assessment of Nutritional Status

The epidemiological approach

There is no single index of nutritional status so assessment is dependent on gathering and correlating data from many sources; by inferential reasoning it is possible to build up an overall picture of the situation.

In the discussion of the ecology of malnutrition it was shown that nutrition is influenced by many factors. The assessment of nutritional status includes an evaluation of these factors and their various interrelationships. This "epidemiological approach" to defining nutritional status has no hard and fast rules, it is still the subject of experimentation and in the present state of knowledge it is not possible as yet, to say which is the most efficient methodology. It may be convenient to start evaluating the availability of food by examining food production in relation to the population and its needs. Further insight into the situation may be gained by determining the food intake or food consumption patterns of samples of the population. Supportive evidence of adequacy of the nutrient intake and the utilization of nutrients may be obtained by examination or measurement of sections of the community who are especially vulnerable to malnutrition. These *vulnerable groups* include growing infants, children, and adolescents and the pregnant and lactating mother who is supplying nutrients for her fetus or suckling infant; it also includes the aged who may, through infirmity, be unable to achieve an adequate nutrient intake.

The methods for evaluating nutritional status and the inferences that can be made from the data are summarized in Table 39 and are now discussed in detail. Students requiring additional information on evaluation of nutritional status should refer to a standard reference on this subject.[1]

Nutritional surveys

In the years following the second World War, international and national agencies encouraged and assisted developing countries to assess the nutritional status of their populations on a systematic and comprehensive basis.

Table 39a   Indirect assessment of nutritional status

Source	Method	Inferences
Agriculture data	Food balance sheets crop calendars Examination of food storage methods.	Per capita food availability. Estimates of food losses and wastage.
Demographic data	Census	Size of "vulnerable groups"
Economic data	Examination of food prices	Ability to purchase adequate diet.
Anthropological Social and Cultural data	Food habits	
	Food customs Food taboos and prejudices	Unavailability of foods
Education		Understanding of food and nutritional needs
Vital Statistics	Morbidity and Mortality experience	Evidence of poor health or death as a result of malnutrition

Table 39b   Direct assessment of nutritional status

Source of Information	Method	Inference
Diet surveys on samples of population	Measurement of food intake	Quantitative and qualitative assessment of intake of food and nutrients
	Analysis of food consumed	Evaluation of effects of processing
Examination of samples of population	Anthropometry	Evidence of achievement of normal growth and development and calorie imbalance
	Clinical	Evidence of malnutrition
	Biochemical	Enzyme changes, alterations in nutrient levels

Many countries seeking bilateral or international aid were advised that it would be unrealistic and wasteful of effort to plan national nutritional programs and services without a clear definition of the nature and extent of the nutritional problems affecting the country, and without an appraisal of its food and nutrition resources. Consequently, nutrition surveys were conducted in developing countries throughout the world as a prelude to the development of national nutrition programs, but because of inadequate evaluation very little is know of the effectiveness of programs which may have resulted. It is quite clear however, that no survey will be of value unless it is part of an overall program in nutrition. As an alternative to using nutrition surveys, some countries have taken note of certain obvious problems, concentrated their programs and services, and postponed the assessment of the overall situation until a more appropriate time. This method of approach may have led to benefits but it will be impossible to measure the effects unless indices for evaluation are "built in" to the program.

Nutrition surveys utilize the epidemiological approach; they also employ direct methods of assessing nutritional status by dietary, clinical, and biochemical means. The methodology for nutritional surveys was first established in 1939;[2] a more recent methodology has been described by the *Interdepartmental Committee on Nutrition for National Development* (ICNND)[3] of the United States. This committee has been responsible for conducting surveys in over 30 countries. Many of the nutrition programs in the world owe their existence to surveys conducted by teams of the ICNND. At first the samples for these surveys were drawn from the armed forces and their families, but later the samples were more representative of the total population and had much greater significance and practical use.

The World Health Organization (WHO) and the *Food and Agriculture Organization* (FAO) with the assistance of the *United Nations Childrens Fund* (UNICEF) have helped many countries to conduct national nutrition surveys. Some of these have become part of on-going surveillances of nutritional status by governments. For example, the Philippines and Iran continue to conduct surveys that provide up-to-date information on nutritional status. They also furnish information on seasonal variations which may not be provided by cross sectional surveys carried out at one time of the year. Nutrition surveys are very expensive, time consuming, and require highly trained personnel that may not be available. They not only provide information but they also generate public and professional interest and encourage involvement of the community. They also serve as a useful medium for training personnel. The nutrition survey in the Sudan for instance, was carried out by a team that moved from province to province where it trained local staff and assisted in the development of a provincial nutrition program.

It is unwise to consider a uniform protocol for procedure because of the variation in availability of financial and manpower resources and varying objectives. It is important that any survey schedule should be prepared according to the particular objectives of the survey and with due regard to other factors such as the educational levels and skills of all of the survey team, facilities for statistical processing, geography, climate, and the characteristics of the population.

A lack of financial resources and professional expertise will prevent surveys from being conducted in many countries for several years. However, it is these poor countries that need the most assistance in defining their nutritional problems. As an interim measure an increased usage is being made of the *Rapid* nutrition survey, which is a practical method of estimating nutritional status.[4] The technique involves the collection of basic information relating to the population and its composition, food, health, morbidity, and mortality. Food habits and consumption patterns and seasonal or yearly trends are examined and related to the theoretical nutritional requirements of the population. A clinical and anthropometric survey of representative groups of the population is also made. Usually the samples are composed of preschool and school children. *Rapid* surveys are based on three assumptions. First, malnutrition is the result of a lack of balance between requirements for, and consumption of, nutrients. Second, it is assumed that clinical signs are reliable indices of malnutrition. Third, it is assumed that subclinical malnutrition may be evaluated through mortality rates for certain diseases such as diarrhea, measles, and whooping cough.

While these assumptions are reasonable, there is the possibility that cases of subclinical malnutrition do not contribute to mortality and that cases of protein malnutrition are missed during the survey. It has been pointed out that the rapidity with which a malnourished child will deteriorate and die decreases the chance of a severe case being detected in a survey of a short duration.[5]

It may not be feasible to embark on a direct assessment of nutritional status that involves an examination of dietary intake, clinical and biochemical appraisal of nutrition, and evaluation of growth. In such cases an indirect assessment may provide useful information from which inferences may be made.

The indirect assessment of nutritional status

Examination of data

Total food production At first sight, increases in total food production may seem satisfactory but the data should be scrutinized to see if the increase in production is associated with an increase in the availability of nutrients for the population. World food production in 1967 showed an increase over 1966, but when the changes in production of the various commodities are examined (see Figure 86) it will be seen that the world production of wheat, citrus fruits and oats declined and the total increase in food production was attributable to increased production of rice, maize, and barley.

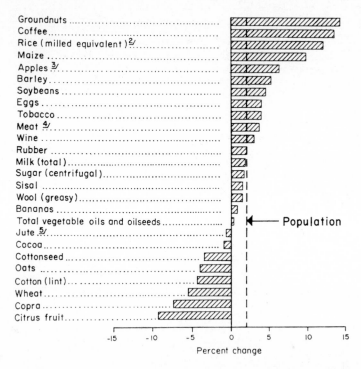

¹ Excluding China (Mainland). – ² Paddy converted at 65 percent. – ³ Excluding the U.S.S.R. and China (Mainland). – ⁴ Beef and veal, mutton and lamb, pork, poultry meat. – ⁵ Including allied fibers.

Figure 86   Changes in world production of main agricultural commodities in 1967 in relation to 1966 (Reproduced from *State of Food and Agriculture* FAO. Rome 1968)

Apart from providing useful data on food available for direct consumption, production data also gives information on potential purchasing power for food. There were considerable increases in cash crops such as coffee and tobacco, and decreases in cotton and copra, but in order to evaluate the significance of these changes, prevailing world market prices should be taken into consideration. A decrease in productivity may be countered by a rise in prices and vice versa. A fall in both production and prices, or a fall in price not countered by an increase in production can be of great economic significance.

Table 40 Total agricultural production: Country, subregional and regional indices

	1952	1953	1954	1955	1956	1957	1958	1959	1960	1961	1962	1963	1964	1965	1966 (Preliminary)
						Indices, average 1952–56=100									
Far east*	92	97	100	104	107	108	112	117	121	126	129	131	135	133	135
Burma	100	97	98	99	106	94	109	116	116	119	130	131	140	133	117
Ceylon	94	94	102	108	102	106	108	111	117	121	128	132	138	133	138
China (Taiwan)	89	101	100	101	108	118	124	123	123	129	128	133	146	159	166
India	90	100	100	104	107	107	111	115	121	125	126	128	131	124	123
Indonesia	93	98	105	102	103	104	108	109	110	109	116	108	117	114	119
Japan	97	86	95	113	110	113	118	117	118	120	129	127	132	133	137
Korea, Rep. of	72	98	110	114	106	116	124	126	125	136	121	136	171	170	184
Malaysia: West Malaysia	94	95	99	106	106	112	112	117	123	131	132	139	141	151	159
Pakistan	99	96	100	99	105	106	104	112	116	119	119	128	127	130	128
Philippines	93	97	99	101	109	114	115	115	123	124	134	138	139	135	151
Thailand	89	106	87	105	113	93	108	114	130	139	146	158	157	167	191
North America	99	99	97	101	103	96	106	107	110	109	112	119	117	119	120
Canada	110	104	79	99	108	92	97	99	107	90	114	127	118	130	144
United States	98	98	99	101	103	99	107	108	110	111	112	118	117	118	118
Oceania	96	97	97	104	106	102	117	119	123	125	133	137	142	136	150
Australia	96	97	97	104	106	100	119	119	124	126	134	139	145	134	153
New Zealand	96	97	98	102	106	107	114	120	122	124	130	131	135	141	145

* Excluding China Mainland.

Source: The State of Food and Agriculture, FAO, 1968

Examination of specific food sources may also provide some useful information. Fish production in 1967 was 5 per cent above that of the previous year; however, the bulk of the increase was due to increased production by Peru, Japan, mainland China, the U. S. S. R., Norway, and South Africa. With the exception of Tunisia and Algeria, which also experienced an increase in fish production, the overall increase could not directly affect those developing countries most in need of high quality protein. The fluctuations in production in different countries of the same region, for example India and Pakistan (see Table 40), may indicate an area where food shortages are likely to occur from time to time.

National Food Balance Sheets Additional information that throws light on the national food situation may be obtained from Food Balance Sheets. As the name implies these give information on the balance of food available to the nation in general. The following equation represents a Food Balance Sheet.

$$\text{Balance} = (T + I + S) - (E + A + N + L + W)$$

where

T = Total food production

I = Imports

S = Food taken from stocks

E = Exports

A = Animal foodstuffs

N = food converted to non-food use

L = Food losses

W = Wastage

Preparing a Food Balance Sheet utilizes data that is crude in nature, and allowances for this must be made during interpretation. For example, supplies can only be assumed to have gone to human consumption and no account can be given of its distribution within the country. They also represent an annual average and cannot give information on seasonal variations (see Table 41).

Food Balance Sheets are relatively cheaper and simpler to prepare than estimates of direct food usage. A Food Balance Sheet is critized frequently because of its scientific inaccuracies; this is a reasonable criticism but governments may be obliged to take whatever information is available.[6]

Per capita availability Total productivity and Food Balance Sheets by themselves do not indicate the per capita availability of food. Increases

Table 41 Food balance sheet for Morocco

Morocco: Food Balance, 1959–61 and Totals for 1956–58 estimated population 11,625,000

Product	Supply					Nonfood use	
	Pro-duction	Imports	Exports	Changes in stocks	Total supply	Seed and waste	Feed
	1,000 m. tons	1,000 m. tons	1,000 m. tons	1,000 m. tons	1,000 m. tons	1,000 m. tons	1,000 m. tons
Barley	925	66	23	...	968	76	160
Wheat	885	178	83	...	980	88	...
Wheat flour	...	16	2	...	14	...	...
Corn	308	...	64	...	244	17	32
orghum and millet	68	...	54	...	14	...	2
Sice	18	2	6	...	14	...	...
Other cereals	*16	...	2	...	14	...	2
Total cereals							
Sugar	...	357	10	...	347	...	...
Potatoes	134	31	57	...	108	11	...
Peanuts	...	8	...	...	8	...	...
Pulses	123	15	11	...	127	12	5
Tomatoes	268	...	125	...	143	20	...
Other vegetables	*154	...	4	...	150	4	...
Citrus fruit	459	...	313	...	146	6	...
Grapes	343	...	1	...	342	15	...
Olives	152	...	...	...	152	...	...
Figs (fresh and dry)	80	...	...	...	80	3	...
Dates	56	2	...	...	58	2	...
Other fruits	*12	11	...	...	23	1	...
Beef and veal	64	...	...	...	64	...	...
Mutton and lamb	34	...	...	...	34	...	...
Other meat	58	...	...	...	58	...	...
Total meat							
Fish	148	1	73	...	76	4	...
Olive oil	22	...	2	+1	19	...	...
Vegetable oils	4	39	...	...	43	...	...
Animal fats	14	12	...	...	26	...	...
Total fats							
Whole milk	532	...	...	...	532	6	...
Cheese	7	3	...	...	10	...	...
Dry milk	...	8	...	...	8	...	...
Total milk and cheese							
Eggs	50	...	3	...	47	...	...
Total consumption 1959–61 1956–58							

Source: *Food Balances for 30 Countries in Africa and West Asia, 1959–61*, U. S. Dept of Agriculture.

	Utilization							
Nonfood use		Supply for food						
					Net			
						Per capita		
Indus-trial	Total	Total gross	Extrac-tion rate	Total	Per year	Calo-ries	Per day	
							Grams protein	Grams fat
1,000 m. tons	1,000 m. tons	1,000 m. tons	Per cent	1,000 m. tons	Kilo-grams	Calo-ries	Grams protein	Grams fat
...	236	732	80	585	50.3	458	15.2	2.5
...	88	892	90	803	69.0	662	22.1	2.8
...	...	14	...	14	1.2	11	0.3	...
...	49	195	97	189	16.3	159	4.2	1.9
...	2	12	85	10	0.9	8	0.2	0.1
...	...	14	70	10	0.9	9	0.2	...
...	2	12	50	6	0.5	5	0.1	0.1
					139.1	1,312	42.3	7.4
...	...	347	93	223	27.8	295	...	...
...	11	97	...	97	8.3	16	0.4	...
...	...	8	...	8	0.7	11	0.5	0.8
...	17	110	...	110	9.5	90	5.8	0.5
...	20	123	...	123	10.6	6	0.3	0.1
...	4	146	...	146	12.5	8	0.5	0.1
...	6	140	...	140	12.0	13	0.3	0.1
305	320	22	...	22	1.9	4	0.1	0.1
146	146	6	...	6	0.5	2	...	0.3
...	3	77	...	77	6.6	20	0.3	0.1
...	2	56	...	56	4.8	37	0.3	0.1
...	1	22	...	22	2.0	3	...	...
					27.8			
...	...	64	...	64	5.5	34	2.2	2.7
...	...	34	...	34	2.9	19	0.9	1.7
...	...	58	...	58	5.0	27	2.7	1.9
					13.4	80	5.8	6.3
...	4	72	...	72	6.2	30	3.4	1.7
...	...	19	...	19	1.6	39	...	4.4
...	...	43	...	43	3.7	90	...	10.1
9	9	17	...	17	1.5	37	...	4.1
					6.8	166	...	18.6
73	79	453	...	453	38.9	81	4.1	4.9
...	...	10	...	10	0.9	10	0.6	0.8
...	...	8	...	8	0.7	7	0.5	0.5
					40.5	98	5.2	6.2
...	...	47	...	47	4.0	16	1.2	1.1
						2,210	66.4	43.5
						2,210	70.3	45.7

Data from *Ecology of Malnutrition in Northern Africa* by Jaques M. May. 1967. Reproduced with permission of Hafner Publishing Company.

in productivity and positive balances in food mean little unless they are related to the needs of the population. Population increases in some developing countries exceed increases in production, so the per capita availability of food may be decreasing in successive years, despite apparent healthy annual production increments. Figure 87 shows the trends in food production and population in developing regions. For all the developing regions, per capita food production stabilized, then, actually fell in 1966.

It may be useful to examine trends for individual food commodities or groups. A further examination of Figure 86 shows that the increases in milk production did not keep pace with the increase in population.

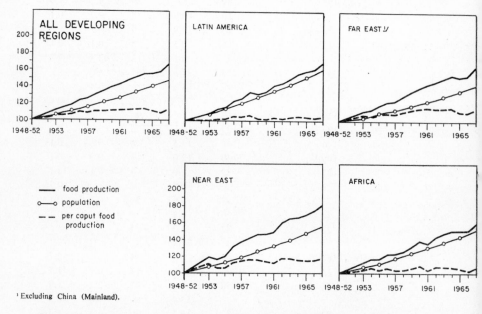

¹ Excluding China (Mainland).

Figure 87   Trends in food production and population in developing regions (Reproduced from *State of Food and Agriculture*, FAO. Rome 1968)

Starchy roots and tubers tend to replace cereals that have a much higher biological value. This trend may become apparent when food production figures are examined over a period of several years. Table 42 shows changes in productivity (and the effects of the poor harvests in India in 1965 and 1966) between 1962 and 1966; the availability of cereals, pulses, and milk has decreased while potato production has increased.

In this, and similar situations, where total calorie or protein availability barely exceeds the estimated requirements, undernutrition is likely. It is

Table 42 Per capital availability of Protein and calories—India 1960–66

India	Cereals	Potatoes	Pulses, Nuts, Seeds	Milk	Protein	Calories
	g/day	g/day	g/day	g/day	g/day	
1960/62	383	29	63	127	49.6	2020
1963/65	380	35	54	117	49.1	1960
1965/66	456	39	41	110	45.4	1810

Source: *State of Food and Agriculture*, FAO. Rome 1968.

even more probable among the poor and where there is maldistribution of food in areas with inadequate natural resources or inclement climatic conditions. When the per capita availability falls below estimated requirements, chronic undernutrition may be expected.

The need to consider quality as well as quantity has already been discussed. A useful measure of quality is obtained from the percentage of calories provided by the protein in the diet. The Protein Calories Per Cent is calculated as follows:

$$\text{Protein Calories } \% = \frac{\text{Protein (grams)} \times 4}{\text{Total calories in diet}}$$

The needs for protein are such that the protein should contribute approximately 4 per cent of the total energy requirements of the reference. If the diet provides less than 4 per cent of its energy in the form of protein, the subject can never consume enough to insure nitrogen balance because the appetite will be satisfied before the required amount of protein is consumed. Table 43 shows that Tanzania's per capita protein calories percent is well above danger level.

The type of staple food available is therefore a good index of whether protein calorie adequacy is being achieved. Table 44 shows the protein calorie per cent of some common staples.

Table 43 Total protein, calories and protein calories Tanzania 1960–1962

Protein	58.1 grams
Calories	2080
Protein cals %	8.9

Source: *State of Food and Agriculture*, FAO. Rome 1968.

Food production and economic growth In 1965 food production failed to increase in developing countries. In 1966 it increased by less than 1 per cent while the populations continued to grow 2.5 per cent per year; as a result

Table 44   Protein calorie percentage of common staples

Food stuff	Protein cals %
Sago flour	0.6
Cassava flour	1.8
Plantains	3.1
Sweet potatoes	5.3
Irish potatoes	10.7
Rice	8.0
Maize flour (whole meal)	10.5
Wheat flour (white)	11.4
Sorghum	11.3

per capita food consumption fell by 4 per cent. Although prospects of recovery were not good, more than half the loss was regained in 1967.[7]

In 22 of 33 individual developing countries reviewed by FAO, food production has been increasing faster than the population. When this is correlated with economic data there are indications that despite the slow pace of economic development, there has been an increase in per capita income. It would seem that economic development is exceeding population increases at last.

Income and food consumption   Research has shown that there is a relationship between per capita income and the amount that is spent on the purchase of foods. This is true for a wide range of countries having different levels of income and economic development, and with widely varying cultures and food habits.[8] The essential connection between economic development and nutritional improvement emphasizes the need to evaluate the former when attempting to determine the nutritional status of a community.

One of the immediate effects of increases in per capita incomes is an increase in demand for purchased food. The increase in demand inevitably exceeds the increase in production of food so food prices move higher in response to the shortage. Part of the newly acquired wealth is absorbed in an increased food budget, but with raised prices the increase in consumption is less than the increase in the budget. The *income elasticity of demand* is a measure of the increase in expenditure of food in response to an increase in income. In developing countries the "income elasticity of demand" is high and might be 0.8. This means that a 10 per cent increase in income would be associated with an 8 per cent increase in expenditure on food. In highly industrialized countries the *income elasticity of demand* may be as low as 0.1.

If high income groups receive an increased income it will have little effect on the total demand for food. If an increase in income benefits the poor who constitute the majority of the population, the increased demand for food will be much greater and may be beyond the resources of the country.[9] This was exemplified in 1968 when food production kept up with demand in only 8 out of 26 countries.

Food and commodity prices   Marketing data should be examined for changes in commodity prices that may indicate a decrease in purchasing power. Table 45 shows food prices were stable or even declining in some countries in 1967. It is unlikely that this trend will continue since fluctuations in market prices are common and dependent on supply and demand, which is constantly changing.

Table 45   Changes in indices of cost of living and retail pood prices, 1967 in relation to 1966, by region

	Europe	North America	Oceania	Latin America	Far East	Near East	Africa	Total
				Number of countries				
Food prices rose faster than cost of living	1	—	2	9	13	5	5	35
Food prices and cost of living rose at about the same rate	6	—	2	6	—	2	8	24
Food prices rose more slowly than cost of living	14	2	—	8	2	1	3	30
Food prices remained stable or declined	1	—	1	6	2	1	10	21

Source: *The State of Food and Agriculture*. FAO. 1968.

In the case of cereals, the type of cereal determines the amplitude of the price fluctuations. Nearly all wheat enters the market before processing but most of the rice that is produced never enters commercial channels. When it does, it is very much more exposed to exploitation because rice is grown by many small farmers who use numerous transporters, processors, storage, and marketing agents. All of these are likely to charge commission which is added to the final retail price. In these circumstances it is inevitable that prices vary from village to village. There is, however, a lack of detailed information concerning these prices which prevents governments from setting national market and price policies. In developed countries there are regulations controlling the grading, standardization, and processing of cereals. The objective of these regulations is to ensure fair trade but in developing countries regulations are rarely found; rice in particular has been neglected. Some attempts to fix prices by government decrees have created a black market where prices are 100–200 per cent higher than official.[10] In some countries, supply and demand has been adjusted through buffer-stocks, and marketing boards have been established to control prices. However, attempts to direct the market through one channel is a hazardous undertaking as it offers the possibilities of developing black markets and encouraging government corruption. Cooperative marketing would appear to be a useful method of establishing prices. It has the distinct advantage that the community is an active participant in the scheme but in India and the Philippines where cooperatives have been tried, market prices have still not stabilized.

Some countries export rice for cash. This certainly helps to maintain the national balance of payments, but it may not bring appropriate benefit or earnings to the producer who may become committed to growing a single crop, thereby becoming dependent on cash.

Food habits and customs   The significance of food habits and customs has already been discussed in Chapter 2; these should be evaluated. By recognizing potentially harmful habits, populations *at risk* may be identified. "Good" food habits should be noted, for it may be possible to use them in subsequent educational programs.

Educational levels   An evaluation of educational levels is important for two reasons. First, it will help to identify groups lacking education and therefore susceptible to the dangers of adopting sophisticated infant feeding practices. It will help also to determine the level at which nutrition education should be directed, in subsequent programs. It will assist in identifying people who may be recruited as assistants in the survey or a subsequent project.

Vital and health statistics   A considerable amount of information can be collected which may give an insight into the characteristics of the population and its life, health, and mortality experience.

The total live population. If a national population census is available, population histograms should be prepared showing the relative proportions of the population in various age groups. This will reveal whether the population is preponderantly young and therefore susceptible to protein calorie malnutrition and childhood deficiencies (see Figure 88), or whether the population is more evenly distributed among all ages (see Figure 89). Trends may be detected by preparing histograms from previous censuses. In local surveys an examination of the characteristics of the population may reveal unusual features in the age structure of the population. Figure 88 relates

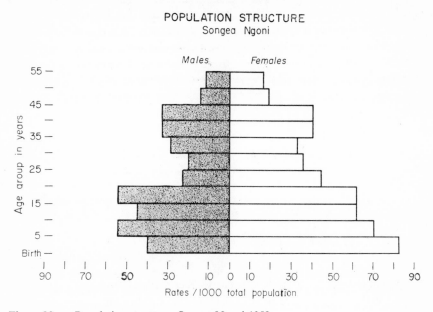

Figure 88   Population structure, Songea Ngoni 1958

to Maposeni (see page 12) and shows the deficit in the male population caused by migration of the men in search of work. The sex ratio at each age group should also be calculated since this may reveal excessive mortality in one of the sexes. In Maposeni it was shown that there was a predominance of females (see Table 46) which raised the possibility that the community was practicing male infanticide.

Births and Deaths   It is useful to establish rates for certain statistics such as birth rates, death rates, and age specific death rates. In highly industrialized countries this presents no problem as it is customary for all births and deaths to be registered. Where registration of births and deaths is not

4*

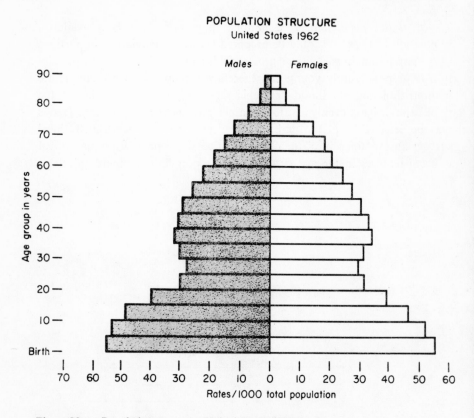

Figure 89   Population structure, United States 1962

compulsory the local church and parish records may provide useful data.
If no reliable records are available then the mother in each household
should be questioned on her reproductive history. The number of pregnancies, the number of abortions, and the number of still and live births are
noted. This should be followed by further questioning on the subsequent
history of each child born alive, cause of death, and the age of occurrence.
From this, it may be possible to gain an insight into death rates by age.

Frequently, problems arise in determining the correct age of children;
in some countries a child becomes one year of age on the arrival of the
traditional New Year. For example, if a child is born in August and the
traditional New Year falls in October, he will assume an age of one year
in that month when he is actually only 2 months of age. Its subsequent
age will always be inflated by 10 months. A local calendar of events may
assist the estimation of the timing of births, deaths, and serious illness.[11]

Table 46 Sex ratio of the Maposeni population
(Males as percentage of females)

By age	
Age group	Sex ratio
Birth–12 months	55.5
13 months – 4 years	45.4
5 years– 9 years	80.7
10 years–14 years	70.8
15 years–19 years	87.3
20 years–24 years	47.1
25 years–29 years	50.0
30 years–34 years	91.6
35 years–39 years	75.0
40 years–44 years	75.0
45 years–49 years	62.2
50 years–54 years	57.2
55 years and over	65.2

Table 47 Natality and mortality experience based on reproductive histories (Rates per 1000 live births)

Country	Mean no. pregnan- cies	Abortion	Stillbirth	Died 0–28 days	0–1 yr	13 mo. to 4 yrs.
Somalia (Rural)	4.0	66	15	106	208	106
Iran (Rural)	5.9	94	9	66	188	255
Iraq (Urban)	4.8	95	36	42	140	60
Tunisia (Urban)	6.3	139	55	97	229	92

Source: Blankhart, D. M.

A reproductive history may be collected in routine questioning at Well Baby clinics or Antenatal clinics.

In areas where health, disease prevalence, or malaria eradication surveys are being conducted, it may be possible for a trained worker to accompany the survey teams to collect this specialized data. Table 47 shows the natality and mortality experience of several Middle East countries based on reproductive histories. Higher rates for stillbirth were observed in the urban areas; the mortality rate in the over-one-year group was probably related to weaning difficulties in the rural areas. On the other hand the high mortality in the under-one-year group in urban Tunisia may reflect infant feeding problems associated with urbanization. In the more advanced countries where accurate records are available it is worth while examining age specific death rates. The most commonly used statistic is the *Infant Mortality Rate (IMR)*. This is the number of deaths occurring under one year of age expressed as a rate for 1000 live births occurring in the same period of time, or

$$\text{Infant Mortality Rate} = \frac{\text{No. of deaths under one year} \times 1000}{\text{No. of live births in the same year}}$$

The Infant Mortality Rate has assumed considerable importance in the evaluation of public health, not only because of its value as an indicator of loss of life, but also because of its close correlation with social conditions (see Table 48). Deaths within the first year have been subdivided further. *Neonatal mortality* refers to deaths under four weeks and *perinatal mortality* relates to stillbirths and deaths under one week. These rates are only valid when the reporting system is sophisticated and reliable. Neonatal mortality reflects deaths in infants who have been debilitated from birth whereas the stillbirth and perinatal mortality is influenced by obstetrical experience.

Table 48 Infant mortality and State income ranking (USA)

States* ranked by per capita income	Per capita income, $, 1965	Infant mortality rate per 1,000 Births, 1965		Nonwhite % of births, 1965
		White	Nonwhite	
1 Connecticut	3,401	20.3	36.9	9.5
2 Delaware	3,392	20.1	40.8	20.4
3 Nevada	3,311	23.7	32.7	11.5
4 Illinois	3,280	21.4	44.5	18.2
5 New York	3,278	20.2	39.5	16.1
46 Tennessee	2,013	23.8	42.0	22.8
47 Alabama	1,910	23.3	43.8	36.6
48 South Carolina	1,846	22.7	43.3	42.1
49 Arkansas	1,845	20.6	37.7	29.9
50 Mississippi	1,608	24.5	54.4	53.6

  * Excludes Washington, D. C.
    Statistical Abstract of the United States, 1967.

Source: Lowe, C. U. *Medical Opinion and Review*. August 1968.

Deaths from hypoglycemia would contribute to the perinatal mortality rate. Infants with intra-uterine growth failure would affect the neonatal mortality.

International comparisons of infant mortality are frequently made (see Table 49). These may not be strictly comparable because of international differences in the form of death certificate, and the way in which the causes of death are tabulated in the different statistical offices. There may be differences between countries in the types of personnel notifying death. In highly industrialized areas all deaths usually have to be certified by a medical attendant. In less developed areas certification may be made by non-medical personnel who may be basing their report on hearsay evidence, perhaps from relatives within the family. There are also differences in the terminology, this is particularly true in the case of stillbirths. In the United Kingdom a stillbirth is defined as "... any child which has issued forth from its mother after the twenty-eighth week of pregnancy and which did not at any time, after being completely expelled, breathe or show any other sign of life". In some countries a child may be classified as a stillbirth even though it may have breathed for some time after delivery.

Declining infant mortality rates are viewed as an index of satisfactory progress in the promotion of child health. However, these rates may be declining for statistical reasons rather than improved health. Failure to register births will reduce the number of live births and the infant mortality rate will be inflated. When registration of births is introduced, the number of reports of live births will increase. This alone will tend to lower the Infant Mortality Rate. Even though there might be a decline in infant mortality This may not mean a significant reduction in deaths from malnutrition. It will be recalled that the kwashiorkor type of protein calorie malnutrition is associated with weaning and prolonged breast feeding. It therefore tends to occur in the second year of life and outside the period over which infant mortality is evaluated.

Child mortality between one and four years of age is extremely important; for whereas the infant mortality rate in a developing country may be 5 to 10 times as great as that in a highly industrialized country, the mortality in children aged one to four years may be 50 to 60 times greater (see Table 50). While the Infant Mortality Rate may be falling, the child mortality rate may be continuing at a high level. Unless the 1–4 year mortality statistic is introduced into standardized reporting procedures, high mortality rates from malnutrition may be overlooked. The form in which this statistic should be presented raises problems. It has been suggested that the 1–4 year mortality should be expressed per 1000 children in the 1–4 year age group.

Table 49 Infant mortality rates for selected countries, 1966

Rank	Country	Rate
1	Sweden (1965)	13.3
2	Netherlands (1965)	14.4
3	Norway (1964)	16.4
4	Finland (1965)	17.6
5	New Zealand	17.7
6	Switzerland (1965)	17.8
7	Australia	18.2
8	Japan (1965)	*18.5*
9	Denmark (1965)	*18.7*
10	United Kingdom	19.6
11	France	*21.7*
12	Eastern Germany	*23.2*
13	United States	*23.4*
14	Canada (1965)	23.6
15	Czechoslovakia	*23.7*
16	Federal Republic of Germany (1965)	*23.8*
17	Belgium (1965)	24.1
18	Singapore	*24.6*
19	Ireland	24.9
20	Union of Soviet Socialist Republics	26.5
21	Austria	*28.1*
22	Bulgaria	*32.2*
23	Greece	33.7
24	Spain	*34.6*
25	Trinidad and Tobago (1964)	35.3
26	Jamaica	35.4
27	Italy (1965)	35.6
28	Hungary (1965)	*38.8*
29	Poland (1965)	41.8
30	Romania	*46.5*
31	Mexico (1965)	60.7
32	El Salvador	*61.7*
33	Portugal	65.0
34	Yugoslavia (1965)	*71.5*
35	Costa Rica (1965)	*75.1*
36	Albania (1965)	86.8
37	Guatemala	*91.5*
38	Chile (1965)	107.1

Source: Chase, H. C. *Pub. Hlth. Rep.* 84: **19**, 1969.

Table 50 Infant and Child mortality rates

	Infant mortality rate per 1000 live births			Mortality rate in children aged 1–4 years per 1000 children of same age		
	1950–52	1960–62	1966	1950–52	1960–62	1966
Sweden	21.0	16.0	13.0*	1.3†	0.9	0.7*
United Kingdom	29.0	22.0	19.0*	1.4†	0.9	0.8*
Argentina	66.8	61.0	59.3	5.0	4.3	2.4
Chile	128.4	117.8	101.9	12.9	8.2	5.0
Colombia	118.0	92.8	81.2	20.4	15.4	10.8
Costa Rica	110.5	66.1	65.0	14.6	7.5	6.0
El Salvador	81.2	72.5	62.1	31.1	17.1	13.5
Guatemala	104.2	89.3	91.4	46.3	32.4	29.5
Jamaica	77.8	49.1	35.4	10.5	6.8	4.7
Mexico	94.5	71.4	62.9	28.6	13.8	10.9
Panama	58.8	51.1	45.0	9.5	7.9	8.0
Peru	102.7	92.9	63.0	19.8	15.7	10.5
Trinidad and Tobago	82.4	42.9	42.8	5.8	5.5	2.0
Uruguay	56.6	44.6	42.7	2.2	1.3	1.3
Venezuela	79.5	52.1	46.7	11.9	5.7	4.9

*1965.   †1950.

Source: Bengoa, J. M., WHO. Chronicle **24**: 553, 1971.

However, this is a difficult figure to obtain in countries where statistics are poor and where populations migrate. If the 1–4 mortality is related to live births, countries with high infant mortality rates have relatively few survivors into the 1–4 year age group and the rates are not comparable with countries with a low infant mortality rate. It has been suggested that the death rate in 1–4 year age group should be related to deaths between the ages of one month and one year. The ratio of these two rates, $\dfrac{1\text{–}4 \text{ year death rate}}{0\text{–}1 \text{ year death rate}}$, has become known as the *Wills Waterlow Index* and is an accepted index of malnutrition.[12]

It should be noted that deaths in the neonatal period should be excluded as they may represent as much as one-third of the total deaths in the first year of life.

National indices of less than 5 per cent may be interpreted as representative of good nutritional conditions, those of 5–9 per cent correspond to an intermediate position, and indices that extend from 10 to as high as 40 per cent are indicative of defective nutritional status.

The Wills Waterlow Index is probably satisfactory in countries where the main mortality from malnutrition is due to kwashiorkor, but with

Table 51   Comparisons of the Wills Waterlow Index in
Industrialized countries

Country	Death rate 0–1 year	Death rate 1–4 years	Wills Waterlow Index %
Norway	16.9	1.0	6
Italy	40.1	1.7	4
Yugoslavia	77.5	4.5	6
New Zealand	19.6	1.1	6

Source: Gordon, J. E., *et al. Amer. J. Med. Sci.* **254**: 121, 1967

increasing urbanization, marasmus is assuming much greater importance. Increases in the death rate in the first year of life from marasmus will increase the denominator of the ratio and reduce its value thereby giving a false impression. Table 51 shows that the ratio is also misleading when applied to some countries in the highly industrialized parts of the world.

Death rates in the second year of life may be the best indicator of childhood mortality from malnutrition and its synergistic interaction with infections.[13] The global range of the second year death rates is shown in Table 52. The second year death rate is undoubtedly a useful index that may be used to evaluate the effects of health and nutrition programs over a period of time.

Causes of death and morbidity

The notification of specific cases of malnutrition would provide excellent data for evaluating nutritional status. In most countries where malnutrition is a problem this is impracticable. There are large sections of the population which have no access to medical care; they are also the deprived sections of the population that are most likely to be suffering from malnutrition. Even though there might be provision of medical care, the clinical awareness of the attending physician plays a large part in the diagnosis. Protein calorie malnutrition has only recently been recognized as a clinical entity and many physicians have not been trained in the recognition of early signs of the disease.

Even though the disease may be recognized, it may not be reportable by law and there may not be an appropriate rubric in the national classification of disease. That the International Classification of Disease did not make provision for the reporting of protein calorie malnutrition until 1965 is an indication of the deficiencies in the reporting system.[14]

Table 52 Second year age-specific death rates, selected countries, by specified years

Annual deaths per 1,000 population, aged 1 year and less than 2 years

−2	2–4	5–9	10–24	25–49	50 or more
Sweden 1963, 0.9	Czechoslovakia 1963, 2.0	Fiji 1963, 5.4	Yugoslavia 1963, 10.6	India, urban Bombay 1961, 25.9	Senegal 1957, 61.0
United Kingdom 1963, 1.5	France 1963, 2.1	Puerto Rico 1960, 5.6	Venezuela 1961, 11.0	Ceylon 1953, 28.5	Guatemala 1963, 62.1
Norway 1963, 1.6	New Zealand 1963, 2.2	Romania 1963, 5.6	Portugal 1960, 16.4	Jordan 1961, 30.0	Guinea 1955, 68.0
Finland 1963, 1.6	Austria 1963, 2.2	Philippines 1960, 5.6	Thailand 1960, 16.4	Mexico 1960, 30.9	India, rural Khanna 1957–59, 72.2
U. S. A. 1963, 1.6	Japan 1963, 2.5	Trinidad 1963, 6.2	Mauritius 1961, 16.9	El Salvador 1961, 31.7	Egypt 1961, 107.0
Australia 1963, 1.6	Greece 1963, 2.8	Singapore 1957, 6.5	Taiwan 1956, 18.5	Grenada 1961, 33.0	Gambia 1949–53, 111.0
Canada 1961, 1.7	Poland 1963, 3.1	Hong Kong 1961, 8.0	Panama 1963, 19.3	St. Kitts 1960–62, 35.9	St. Vincent 1960–62, 147.6
Israel 1963, 1.7	Italy 1963, 3.2	Barbados 1960–62, 8.7	Antigua 1961–63, 21.1		
Netherlands 1960, 1.7	Hungary 1963, 3.2		Chile 1960, 24.3		
Scotland 1963, 1.8	Spain 1961, 3.6				

Source: Gordon, J. E. *et al. Am. Jour. Med. Sci.* **254**: 129, 1967.

The clinical picture of protein calorie malnutrition is varied; the disease may terminate in a respiratory, cardiac, or gastro-intestinal crisis. The final crisis may be reported as the immediate cause of death, whereas the underlying malnutrition may have been the actual cause of the fatality. The extent to which malnutrition may be hidden in mortality and morbidity statistics may be judged from studies in Guatemala 15 (see Table 53). The synergism between malnutrition and infection has already been discussed, and the significance of high prevalence rates for acute diarrheal disease and attack rates emphasized.

Table 53 Registered and clinical cause of death in Guatemalan children

Cause	Source of information	
	Civil Register	INCAP Study
Respiratory infections	35	42
Infections, whooping cough	11	14
intestinal parasites	12	17
Other causes		
Kwashiorkor	0	40
Others	1	3
III defined disease	41	17

Source: Behar, M., Ascoli, W., Scrimshaw, N. S., WHO. Bulletin **19:** 1093, 1958.

Direct assessment of nutritional status

The direct assessment of nutritional status of communities

Diet and food consumption surveys   These are time consuming, costly, laborious, and they require skilled personnel. In addition to supplying data on food intake, they should also provide social, cultural, and economic information which may help to define the ecology of the food and diet practices of the population. They should always be considered as part of a coordinated national effort to improve nutrition. The salient points of food consumption surveys will now be reviewed; for further information, the reader is referred to one of the standard publications on this subject.[16,17]

National food consumption surveys require extensive planning since they involve numerous small surveys in areas selected to represent different geographical, economic, and cultural conditions, seasonal variations, and economic cycles.

Preliminary planning A very important part of the planning is statistical. The survey design should follow recognized sampling principles to ensure that the results are truly representative of the country and its population. It is possible that other national surveys such as malaria prevalence surveys, or surveys of environmental health, might have recorded and designated census tracts and samples. The availability of such information may determine whether the sample is systematically selected at random, or stratified. If problems are already known the sample may be purposive.

Considerable organization and coordination of effort is required, for the survey may involve workers from many disciplines. It is often convenient for the planning and execution of the survey to be in the charge of a national committee composed of senior officials from the departments or ministeries responsible for the survey. Usually these include the Department of Agriculture, Department of Health, Bureau of Statistics. They should secure adequate financing for the duration of the project; too many surveys in the past have not been completed because of lack of foresight, planning and funding. Once the survey has commenced, the committee should monitor progress continuously and amend its direction or methodology as required. From time to time, the data should be interpreted and used as a basis for program planning. If a specific nutritional problem is discovered in a community, remedial action may be called for immediately.

After the survey area or population has been selected, several important preliminary steps should be taken before the team enters the survey area.

First, all possible efforts should be made to inform the community of the objectives of the survey and to solicit their collaboration. The assistance of prominent local citizens, the specialized skills and knowledge of politicians, community leaders and anthropologists, may be required at this stage.

During the preliminary phases and while the collaboration of the community is being secured, other data should be collected which will supplement or clarify information obtained in the diet survey and contribute to an understanding of the overall epidemiology of the situation. For example, information on traditional taboos, prejudices, beliefs, and attitudes towards food, information on agricultural methods, land tenure, housing, clothing, religion, and disease patterns may also be used to support the dietary data and add to the total picture.

It is informative to define and describe the food year by means of a *crop calender*. This is prepared by noting the months of the year when individual food items are available. These times are then plotted over a period of thirteen months. The *hungry months* when food supplies are limited in variety and quality may become apparent. The time of the survey can then be related to food availability. It may be desirable to postpone a survey if it is scheduled during a hungry month, or during a time of intense activity when householders and farmers are preoccupied with important work such as planting or harvesting.

Figure 90 is a crop calender for a rural community in East Africa showing the limitations in food supplies during the months of January and February.

Figure 90   Crop Calender. Note the limited food resources in January and February, the *hungry months*.

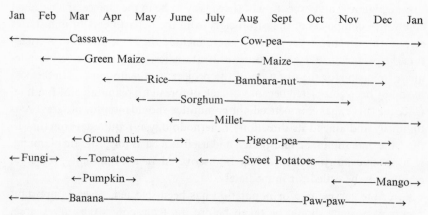

Equipment and supplies   Before embarking on a survey, the team should ensure that it has the necessary basic equipment and supplies. It should also confirm that it can use this equipment. The calculation of food and nutrient intake requires that the food be weighed; in addition the height and weight of the population should be measured. This necessitates the acquisition of simple but reliable weighing machines and the skills to use them. Unfortunately it is assumed that most weighing scales are accurate and that weighing techniques are infallible. Most scales have a small "built-in" error and some have serious design faults that cause inaccurate measurements. The errors do not end at this point however, for the measurer can make serious errors when recording the data.

A preliminary evaluation of techniques, and their ability to produce valid and reproducible height and weight data, is an essential preliminary procedure to any survey.

Training   All surveys require the transfer of information from the community, the household, or an individual, to an investigator. As the conclusions relating to food intake depend on the reports and measurement of food consumed, the importance of training competent and skilled field workers who are acceptable to the community, cannot be overemphasized. The training sessions in weighing food should also be supplemented by training in interviewing, and practice in collecting information on food habits. The collection of dietary data not only requires a knowledge of local food habits, but also an understanding of the principles of nutrition. A compromise may have to be reached between the use of persons educated and not conversant in local food habits, and locally knowledgeable people who may be lacking a proper educational background.

Interviewing Much of the accuracy and validity of food consumption surveys depends on human qualities. For example, the personality of the field worker may determine whether information is readily given or withheld. A conciliatory attitude may cause the householder to paint a more rosy picture of her food intake than actually exists. Disharmony among the field workers may disturb the community who may lose interest and report inaccurately. Even the way questions are posed may determine the answer. For example, one interviewer may present a question that elicits a positive answer, while another asking the same question in a different way may be given a negative type of answer. The questionnaire should be constructed so that all questions are phrased similarly.

The data on food consumption has to be related to the consumer. This entails recording the characteristics of the sample including age, relation to the head of the household, number in family, sex, education, income, marital and physiological status. Questioning on these matters may be extremely difficult. An apparently innocent question may incite offence or it may so encroach on an individual's personal sensitivities that answers may be inaccurate or even refused. Care, tact, and persistence are required, and a certain amount of cross-checking of answers may be needed to ensure that the record is as accurate as possible.

Standards of Measurement The collection of the food record is of prime importance and every effort has to be made to ensure that measurements are accurate; problems arise because different units of measure may be used in different locations. The units need to be clearly defined and those such as a "hand" or a "bunch" have to be reduced to a standard unit of weight or volume. Even in highly sophisticated countries some units are used that are peculiar to localities; for example, the peck is a common measure in the midwest of the United States, a gill is a measure of volume in certain parts of England and Scotland. In the absence of an official measure, it may be customary to cut cheese or foods of a similar consistency to the size of a local cigarette packet. Sometimes a tobacco tin is used to measure sugar or salt. The weight or volume of such containers should be measured in standard units.

If cooked foods are brought for weighing in a cooking utensil, the total weights of the food and the utensil are measured. In order to determine the weight of the food, a similar empty container is weighed and this amount is then deducted from the whole.

Describing the food Foods need to be carefully described and recorded both in its raw and cooked state. For example, milk should be qualified by a further note on whether it is skimmed or whole. It should be noted whether canned fish was packed in oil, sauce, or water. The extraction rates of cereals have to be determined since milling is an important determinant of nutritive value. Local vegetables frequently present problems, for many vegetables may not be recognized by interviewers strange to an area. Particular care has to be taken to ensure that the local name of all foods of this nature is recorded so it may be possible, at a later date, to trace the correct botanical designation.

The edible portion of the food frequently differs from the cooked portion so that note has to be made of whether a fruit was peeled or whether rind or skin was removed before cooking.

Food prices The monetary cost of food should be recorded. Prices in a village without a market may differ from one where food is bought, sold, or exchanged. Even in industrialized countries, there is a marked difference between the prices in the inner city "supermarkets" and the more affluent suburbs. Some foods such as flavorings, spices, green leaves, are produced and consumed on the homestead and may never be bought or sold; this adds to the difficulties of evaluating family budgets. It is useful to ascertain how long a person would have to work as a laborer or manual worker in order to buy a fixed quantity of bone-free meat, or milk. This simple procedure allows comparison to be made between areas differing widely in wages and food prices.

Food records The data can be recorded in a variety of ways. A record can begin at any meal; a note is made of the menu, its ingredients, food which is not consumed, the numbers of family present and the numbers of visitors. The record should continue for at least a week to reveal day to day variations in food consumption. The variations may be related to the availability of money for food purchases (more money is likely to be available the day after pay day than the day before) or religious customs.

As an alternative, an inventory of food consumed can be prepared. All the food in the household is measured at the beginning of the survey period. Subsequently, all food purchased, wasted, or given away, and the food remaining in the household at the end of the survey is measured. From this, it is possible to calculate the daily average consumption of food of the household. For those members of the family who eat away from home, this method may still be used, but every absence should be recorded. Feast and fasts complicate diet records, therefore diet inquiries should avoid

Table 54   Changes in food consumption 1955–1965. United States Households

Food	Per cent change in household consumption from 1955 to 1965			
	Northeast	North Central	South	West
Increases				
Nonfat dry milk	140	100	138	129
Salad, cooking oils	92	100	117	19
Bakery products except bread	64	66	79	48
Beef	30	22	56	14
Chicken	20	27	21	37
Commercially frozen:				
Potatoes	150	375	1,300	250
Vegetables	30	21	62	25
Potato chips, sticks	140	60	83	46
Fresh fruit juice	381	267	167	575
Soft drinks	86	77	68	96
Fruit made drink, punch, nectar	1,036	764	756	457
Peanut butter	50	57	67	45
Decreases				
Fresh fluid milk	12	18	23	24
Evaporated milk	23	42	40	46
Butter	26	34	54	40
Shortening	30	35	37	49
Flour	31	31	50	42
Sugar	7	20	15	22
Fresh white potatoes	18	18	15	25
Fresh vegetables	18	17	19	15
Fruit:				
Fresh	5	21	11	15
Commercially frozen	64	50	43	38

Source: Household Food Consumption Survey. Report No. 2. U. S. D. A. 1968.

these times if possible. For example, the dates of the *Moslem* 28-day fast of *Ramadhan* are usually known well in advance, and they should be determined by preliminary inquiries. Family feasts are less predictable and are liable to introduce bias into the inquiry for they frequently contain foods of high nutritive value. Again it should be remembered that the family survey does not take into account distribution of food within the family. This is of course, particularly unfortunate because the infant, child, and mother carry an increased risk of malnutrition.

It is obvious that the collection of data is fraught with pitfalls but with care and the use of skilled techniques, reliable information can be obtained. Tables 54, 55, and 56 show some of the results of the last decennial Household Food Consumption Survey in the United States. The survey in 1965 revealed changes in consumption patterns compared with 1955. Differences were also noted in intakes between geographical regions, income levels, and urban and rural areas. At first the nutritional significances of these differences may not be apparent but when other sources of information are examined as well, the inconsistencies in intakes may have much more meaning. It will be noted for example, that less fruit is consumed in the south of the United States, than in the other three regions. This observation should be linked with the low serum vitamin C levels noted in the National Nutrition Survey (see page 43).

Table 55   Regional differences in food consumption, United States

		Per person per week			
Food group		Northeast	North Central	South	West
Milk, cream, cheese (calcium equivalent)	qt	4.26	4.20	3.74	4.23
Fats, oils	lb	0.75	0.78	0.94	0.77
Flour, cereal	lb	1.08	1.20	1.95	1.31
Bakery products	lb	2.58	2.38	2.13	2.20
Meat, poultry, fish	lb	4.62	4.68	4.48	4.58
Eggs	doz	0.49	0.55	0.61	0.58
Sugar, sweets	lb	0.97	1.08	1.33	1.01
Potatoes, sweetpotatoes	lb	1.68	1.88	1.48	1.39
Other vegetables	lb	3.50	3.33	3.81	3.73
Fruit	lb	4.18	3.76	3.20	4.01
Soup, other mixtures	lb	0.68	0.63	0.46	0.68

Source: Household Food Consumption Survey 1965–66. Report No. 2. U. S. D. A. 1968.

Table 56 Food consumption in urban and rural areas, United States

| Selected foods | Per person per week | | | |
| | North* | | South | |
	Urban	Farm	Urban	Farm
Urban families used more	Pounds	Pounds	Pounds	Pounds
Vegetables:				
Commercially canned	0.94	0.75	0.94	0.50
Commercially frozen	0.22	0.11	0.19	0.05
Fruit juice	0.82	0.46	0.66	0.36
Bakery products	2.43	2.18	2.26	1.67
Soups, sauces, other mixtures	0.51	0.34	0.41	0.17
Farm families used more				
Lard, vegetable fat	0.10	0.24	0.24	0.49
Fresh white potatoes	1.33	2.32	1.20	1.56
Flour	0.24	0.95	0.49	1.49
Sugar	0.56	1.10	0.78	1.15

* Northeast, North Central, and West.

Source: Household Food Consumption Survey 1965–66. Report No. 2. U. S. D. A. 1968.

Because of a lack of resources, it may not be possible to conduct a food consumption survey and the investigator may have to revert to other kinds of quantitative or qualitative inquiry.

Weekly food diaries Individuals may keep a record of food they consume over a period of a week. The recorder needs careful briefing, orientation, and preparation, and it is essential that all persons selected are both literate and conscientious enough to make faithful records of all that is eaten or imbibed. The daily food consumption is computed from the weeks record.

When data from several areas are compared it may be possible to discern significant differences in food consumption patterns. Table 57 shows the differences in staples, meat consumption, and green leaves in the various localities in Nigeria. Where it is not possible to collect data over prolonged periods, other techniques involving an assessment of intake over shorter periods of time must be used.

24-hour recall

This is an abbreviated survey method. The interviewer asks the householder for information on all foods consumed during the previous 24 hours; it

5*

Table 57 Average diets of six Nigerian villages based on means of four seasons in each locality, expressed in grams edible portion per head per day*

Foodstuff	Igun 1960–61	Abebe-yun 1960–61	Vodni Oct. '61 (Moslems)	Vodni Oct. '61 (Non-Moslems)	Maku 1962–63	Idembia 1962–63	Adiasim 1962–63
Yams: fresh	581	700	—	16	367	260	186
Irish potatoes			15	96			
Sweet potatoes			—	—			
Cocoyams: fresh	—	14	43	84	349	104	125
Plantains: fresh	131	188	—	—			24
Cassava: fresh	276	330	—	—	426	693	820
Maize: dry grain	14	29	—	70	5	—	10
debranned meal	—	—	249	315	—	—	1
refined meal	55	35	—	—	—	—	—
Millet: whole meal	—	—	279	110	—	—	—
Sorghum: whole meal	—	—	82	—	—	—	—
Acha: dry grain	—	—	29	54	—	—	—
Rice: dry grain	16	6	30	—	1	1	1
Wheat: bread	3	2	—	—	—	—	—
Cowpeas: dry beans	48	45	—	6	19	—	7
Wild beans					8	9	2
Locust beans: fermented	11	10	19	14	1	—	—
Melon seeds: dry	3	3	—	—	1	1	7
Benniseed						5	
Groundnuts						5	
Okra fruits: fresh	19	19	36	26	18	9	8
Leafy vegetables: fresh	26	17	14	26	142	16	25
Tomatoes, egg plants	4	5	3	1	15	∅	1
Chilies: fresh	36	23	7	1	24		6
Onions: fresh	1	5	1	6	1		
Meat and bone scraps: fresh	15	14		18	7	9	3
Cow hide: soaked	1	2	—	—			
Fish with bones: dry	3	7	—	—	6	9	10
Crayfish and some insects	1	2		—	3	7	7
Cow's milk: fresh whole	1	1	170	4	—	—	—
Snails: fresh	1	—	—	—	1		—
Red palm oil	19	30	32	29	35	10	14
Groundnut oil			2	—			
Butter: unclarified			4	—			
Kola seeds	12	3	18	2	—	—	—
Pachilobus pulp	—	—	—	—	—	—	5
Tetracarpidium seeds	8	1	—	—	—	—	—

Table 57 *(cont.)*

Foodstuff	Igun 1960-61	Abebe yun 1960-61	Vodni Oct. '61 (Mos-lems)	Vodni Oct. '61 (Non-(Mos-lems)	Maku 1962-63	Idembia 1962–63	Adiasim 1962–63
Palm wine and cereal beer	175	153	—	441	132	46	169
Tea drink	1	1	—	11	—	—	—
Sugar: refined	1	1	16	1	—	—	—
Cooking salt	3	4	6	5	10	7	5
Canarium seed	—	—	—	9	—	—	—
Papaw		∅				—	1
Pumpkin fruit	—	—	—	—	—	1	7
Oranges: juice	—					—	1
Copra: fresh	—	—	—	—	1	—	∅

* In the body of the table, blank spaces mean no data available, dashes indicate zero, and ∅ means trace, which is much less than 1.

Source: Dema, I. S. *Nutrition in Relation to Agricultural Production.* FAO., Rome. 1965.

Table 58 Frequency of intake of foods in Potawotami Indians

Food group	Adults (Mean consumption)		School children (Mean consumption)		Preschool children (Mean consumption)	
	July	April	July	April	July	April
Meat	1.54	1.34	1.08	1.42	0.70	0.90
Total dairy products	1.44	2.45*	1.75	1.90	2.50	2.70
Fresh milk	0.00	0.10	0.36	0.79*	0.70	1.40
Canned milk	1.25	2.34*	1.13	1.01	1.40	1.10
Eggs	0.48	0.77	0.05	0.29	0.60	0.30
Legumes	0.14	0.05	0.00	0.29	0.20	0.20
Bread, cereal	3.36	3.79	3.84	3.74	3.60	4.10*
Potatoes	1.34	0.91	1.32	1.44	1.10	1.20
Fruits and vegetables	1.49	0.77*	0.91	1.46*	1.10	1.00
Snacks and desserts	2.98	2.88	2.14	1.32*	1.30	1.90
Fats	3.07	2.74	3.24	2.95	2.50	2.10

* Significant at 0.05 level

Source: Larkin, F. A., Sandretto, A. M., *J. Home Ec.* **62:** 387, 1970.

requires skilled and careful interviewing techniques. Food or food models should be used for estimating standard portion sizes. It is possible to obtain a reasonably accurate estimate of not only the food pattern, but also the quantity of foods consumed.[18]

It has been found that there is a good correlation between the quantity and frequency of food eaten.[19] The frequency of consumption of food can be determined with relative ease and an increasing use is being made of this method to evaluate diets. The technique requires an interviewer to question each household on items consumed during the previous 24 hours. When information from several households is pooled, it is possible to compare the intakes of different populations, or groups within a population. Table 58 shows seasonal variations in food consumption patterns of Potawotami Indians in Northern Michigan. The impact of the availability of school meals on the consumption of fresh milk and fresh fruits in April, can also be noted. The frequency of intake of foods for a group can also be compared with recommended intakes. Table 59 shows that the intake of green leafy or yellow vegetables by university athletes did not meet recommendations.

The diets of school children can be evaluated by a modification of this method. Children in the fourth grade may be interviewed to determine

Table 59 Food frequencies (University Athletes)

Foods	Mean intake and recommended intake by food groups	
	Mean intake per day	Recommended intake per day
Bread	4.1	3.0 or more
Breakfast cereal, pasta	0.9	
Milk	2.3	2.0
Milk in other foods	0.4	
Ice Cream	0.4	
Citrus fruit	1.0	1.0
Green leafy or yellow vegetables	0.1	1.0
Other fruits and juices	0.6	2.0
Other vegetables	1.1	
Luncheon and filled meat	0.4	2.0
Other meat, fish, poultry	2.1	
Eggs	0.6	
Legumes, nuts, peanut butter	0.3	
Cakes, cookies, pie, donut, sweet rolls	1.3	no recommendation

Source: Larkin, F. A., Davis, B., Robson, J. R. K.

the frequency of consumption of various items in their diet. The technique requires care but by questioning the children privately, and one by one, a general idea of the food pattern of the community may be obtained. In remote and deprived areas where the diet is monotonous and limited in variety, children whose diet patterns differ from the rest of the village can be detected readily. Table 60 shows the pattern of intake of African school children. The consumption of refined cereal flours and the lack of good quality protein can be responsible for protein calorie malnutrition and deficiency of vitamins of the B group. The diet of these school children follows this pattern. The use of condensed milk, the frequent use of sugar and carbonated beverages, are typical of the changes that take place in populations that are becoming urbanized.

Table 60 Frequency of consumption of foods (African School Children)

Food group	Mean frequency per day
Whole meal flours	0
Refined flours and polished rice	2.4
Starchy roots, fruits	0.3
Legumes	0.9
Vegetables ⎰dark green leaves	0.7
Vegetables ⎱pale green leaves and mixed	0.3
Fruits ⎰citrus	0.2
Fruits ⎱others	1.4
Animal products ⎰meat, poultry	0.4
Animal products ⎱fish	0.8
Milk ⎰fresh cows	0
Milk ⎱other fresh milk	0
Milk ⎱condensed	1.8
Syrup, sugar	2.7
Oils and fats	0.5
Beverages—soft drinks	1.2

Source: Robson, J. R. K.

Social Science techniques

Attempts are now being made to evaluate diets by techniques developed in the Social Sciences.[20] Questionnaires are used to collect data on frequency of food consumption, number of meals, social variables such as the level of education of various members of the household, occupation, and housing conditions. Various degrees of complexity of living can be defined for the community, and correlations can be made between certain types of housing, kitchen facilities, occupations, education, and diet patterns. By the use of statistical procedures, including rank correlations and comparisons of variables, it is possible to assign a rank to a household with respect to diet complexity. With further development, it may be possible to evaluate nutritional status by these techniques.

Interpretation of data

The indirect assessment of nutritional status by means of Food Balance Sheets, food productivity, and market surveys provide information on the per capita daily availability of food. A per capita daily intake of food can be obtained from food consumption surveys. Despite the inaccuracies of these techniques it is useful nevertheless to transform per capita food intakes into per capita nutrient intakes. *Food Composition Tables* giving the content of a variety of nutrients per unit weight in various food items are used. Usually the tables give values for protein, calories, water, fat, vitamins, and sometimes minerals. Some of the food tables are intended for use in industrialized countries.[21] Others are used in the tropics.[22] Many countries are producing their own food composition tables that contain information on foodstuffs grown and prepared in their own environment. More detailed analyses of amino acids or other nutrients of importance in dietary work are also available.[23,24]

There are unfortunately many pitfalls in using food composition tables. They should be used with caution because they are frequently abbreviated and may lack an adequate explanation of how they were prepared.

Food composition tables

Interest in the composition of food dates back to pre-Christianity. Hippocrates for example, taught that there was only one universal nutrient, but research over hundreds of years has greatly enlarged the field of knowledge. Early food tables were concerned with the energy producing components of food, namely crude fat, crude protein, carbohydrate, ash, and water. Energy was expressed as calories.

An examination of food composition tables brings to light many factors influencing the validity of the data. No table is suitable for the accurate estimation of individual diets but they are useful in calculating the approximate value of diets of families, communities, or national populations.

Types of food tables   One kind of food table contains data compiled in one laboratory by a particular group of workers. These data are only accurate for the samples analyzed at that time, so that the extreme accuracy often shown in these tables may be misleading. Other food composition tables have been compiled from analyses of food made in many laboratories throughout the world. In some instances, the editors have selected figures which were believed to be representative of a large number of analyses; however, an average value obtained in this way may still be weighted by an inaccurate figure. Sometimes these averages are based on very few analyses and the results may be far from representative. The third type of food composition table is found in textbooks and manuals which may have been compiled from other tables.

Compilation of Food Tables

Conversion factors   The protein content of food is determined indirectly by ascertaining the amount of nitrogen present. Protein is assumed to have a nitrogen content of 16 per cent so the factor of 6.25 is used to convert the nitrogen to protein. In actual fact, not all proteins have the same nitrogen content so where strict accuracy is required, conversion factors appropriate for each food should be used. Some of the conversion factors are shown in Table 61.

Table 61   Conversion factors for protein content of foods

Food	Conversion factor
Whole Wheat	5.83
Low extraction wheat flour	5.70
Rice	5.46
Sorghum	6.25
Soya beans	5.71
Groundnuts	5.46
Other legumes	6.25
Milk	6.25

The list of foods for which conversion factors are known is incomplete; where the value is unknown, the factor 6.25 is used.

The caloric value of food is determined by physical calorimetry. The value obtained by this method does not represent however, the calorific value of the food to the human body. Some of the food material may not be digested or absorbed, or absorbed materials may not be completely oxidized. Conversion factors that take this into account are applied to three nutrients, protein, carbohydrate, and fat, to give an approximate estimate of their calorific value. The figures ased are 4 Calories per gram of protein,

4 Calories per gram of carbohydrate, and 9 Calories per gram of fat. However, when individual diets are evaluated, more precise factors should be applied. It has been suggested that more appropriate factors would be 3.75 Calories for the heat of combustion of one gram of glucose and other monosaccharides, 4.1 Calories per gram of protein, 9.3 Calories per gram of fat, and 7.0 Calories per gram of alcohol.[25] In practice, different factors are used in different countries. Even within one country the method used may vary from one laboratory to another and individual workers may use different methods from time to time.

The methods used to determine the amount of carbohydrate in a diet are the cause of other errors. In some instances it is not always feasible to estimate the carbohydrate present, and the carbohydrate content is determined *by difference*. In this method the carbohydrate is calculated by adding the percentages of water, protein, fat and ash; this total is then subtracted from 100. The remainder corresponds approximately to the percentage of total carbohydrate but it also includes fiber that is not utilized by the body. In some tables the fiber content is determined separately and subtracted from the total carbohydrate; this gives the *available carbohydrate*.

Food composition tables only give the amounts of calcium, iron, phosphorus, and other nutrients actually present in the food. The quantity absorbed depends on a variety of individual circumstances and also on the interactions of other food ingested at the same time. The absorption of calcium, for example, seems to depend on individual needs for this mineral.[26] It also depends on the presence of phytic or oxalic acid present in the diet. Attempts have been made to make allowances for this and tables giving the phytic acid content of foods are available, but even these values are probably invalid as the phytic acid content of food is affected by processing.[27]

Other inaccuracies arise because of variations in the composition in different samples of a food source, variations in composition in different parts of a single food source, and the effects of storage, processing, and preparation, and cooking of the food.

Variations in food composition Variations in the fat content of meat and fish have already been mentioned. Large variations are also found in the vegetable kingdom. There is evidence that the composition of plant food depends on its botanical variety, and the climatic and topographical conditions under which the food is grown.

Table 62 shows the differences in composition in sweet potatoes grown in New Guinea Highlands and Lowlands.

Table 62 Nutrient content of sweet potatoes

Source	Crude protein (%)	Real protein (%)
New Guinea Highlands	0.5–1.3	82.0
New Guinea Lowlands	3.5	71.0

Source: Oomen, H. A. P. C., *Trop. Geog. Med.* **13**: 321, 1961.

Table 63 Variations in the ascorbic acid content of oranges

Type of orange	Average ascorbic acid mg/100 gm of juice
Navel, California-grown	61
Valencia, grown in:	
California	49
Florida	37

Source: Bernice K. Watt, U. S. D. A., Washington, D. C.

Differences observed in the average content of ascorbic acid in oranges, associated with variety and location, are illustrated in Table 63.

In animal foods, differences in nutrient composition may occur when analyses are made on food in different raw states (fresh or dried). Sometimes it is not specified whether an analysis has been made on the whole carcass or on flesh alone. The composition of fish and meat and their products depends on the type of animal, its age, diet, environment, the season of the year, and its activity before slaughter. A small change in the proportions of fat and bone can make a great difference in the content of all the nutrients. In the United States, studies of poultry over a period of time have shown differences in nutritive content associated with changes in breeding, feeding, and management practices. Data on composition that were suitable for young chickens twenty to forty years ago no longer apply to the chickens now marketed in the USA. The present day chickens are very much younger, they have grown faster, their body composition now shows a 10 per cent increase in water, a 50 per cent reduction in fat, and a caloric value about 30 per cent less than the young chicken of similar weight of the earlier period.

Identification of samples Some food varieties may resemble one another in appearance but they may differ botanically. Samples of roots and tubers may inadvertently be assigned to the wrong category. This would introduce errors into the analyses of that particular group of foods. For example, a yam mistaken for a sweet potato would be credited with 20 per cent more calories.

Moisture content   A change in moisture content will affect the concentration of all nutrients. Table 64 shows the variation in reports of the protein and moisture in sorghum.

Table 64   Variations in the water and protein content of Sorghum

Source	Water (%)	Protein (%)
U. S. D. A. Handbook 8	11.0	11.0
Medical Research Council, Report No. 302	12.0	10.0
American University Beirut Publication No. 20	10.0	8.8
Sudan Food Values (Henry, A. J.)	5.7	14.2

Table 65   Variations in the protein and lysine content of sorghum varieties

Variety	Protein % (Nx 6.25)	Lysine (% of protein)
Conspituum	8.61	1.29
Tall White Kaffir	12.06	1.29
Cernum	17.68	2.13

Source: Virpoksha, T. K., Sastry, L. V. S., *Ag. Food Chem.* **16**: 99, 1968.

Within a single species there may be considerable variations which are independent of moisture content. This may be important when hybrids are bred for protein (see Table 65). Variations have also been observed in the protein and amino acid content of sorghum hybrids grown in different locations.[28]

Storage   The depreciation of food under storage conditions has been discussed in Chapter 2. In addition, the nutrient value of the food may also decrease. It has been noted that losses of vitamin C ranging between 47 and 71 per cent may occur in stored potatoes.[29] Losses are not confined to raw foods, since the vitamins in canned food may be destroyed also with the passage of time (see Table 66).

Table 66   Losses of ascorbic acid in stored canned fruit juices

Fruit Juice	Percentage loss over 10 months
Pineapple—grapefruit	25.8
Pineapple—pear	31.0
Orange—apricot	36.0

Source: Brody, A. L., Bedrosian, K. *Food Technology*, **15**: 367, 1961.

Effects of processing and preparation   Analyses of food may have been made on the whole item *as purchased*. However, in preparing the food for consumption the peel or rind, or the core of the food may be removed. Sometimes the outer layer of a peeled food is an area particularly rich in vitamins (see Table 67).

Table 67   Distribution of ascorbic acid across the tuber of yams

Site	Ascorbic acid content (mg/100 g)
Immediately under the skin	12.0
Midway between skin and axis	11.2
At axis	10.1

Source: Coursey, D. G., Aidoo, A., *J. Sci., Food, Agric.*, **17**: 447, 1966.

If the food information is to be *translated* accurately, care should be taken to ensure that the food composition table supplying the data is furnishing information on the part that has been consumed. Large errors can creep into *translations* if this precaution is not taken. The carotene content on cabbages may be based on whole cabbage which includes the outer green leaves. These are the richest source of carotene but most householders remove the outer leaves before cooking. Milling and pounding of cereals removes part of the germ. In so doing, the protein content of the cereals is reduced (see Table 68).

Washing food may reduce the content of the water-soluble vitamins. Similarly, soaking food and discarding the water will also mean a loss of vitamins. Table 69 shows the losses of water-soluble vitamins during the preparation of rice.

Important amino acids may be destroyed during the heat treatment of milk, a necessary procedure in infant formula preparation (see Table 70).

Table 68 Effects of Milling on protein content of wheat flours

Extraction Rate Percentage	English Wheat % Protein (Nx 6.25)	Manitoba Wheat % Protein (Nx 6.25)
100 (Whole wheat)	9.75	14.93
85	9.37	14.87
80	9.00	14.50
75	8.75	14.31
70	8.68	14.00
"Patent" flour	8.37	12.93

Source: McCance, R. A., Widdowson, E. M. Special Report, No. **297**, 1967.

Table 69 Effect of washing on vitamins in rice

	Thiamine			Riboflavin			Nicotinic acid		
	Before Washing μg/g	After Washing μg/g	Percent Loss	Before Washing μg/g	After Washing μg/g	Per cent Loss	Before Washing μg/g	After Washing μg/g	Per cent Loss
Raw lightly milled	2.6	2.0	15	0.50	0.45	10	25	20	20
Raw highly milled	0.9	0.5	44	0.25	0.20	20	20	15	25

Source: *Tropical Nutrition and Dietetics* by Nicholls, L., Sinclair, H. M., Jelliffe, D. B., 4th Edition, 1961.

Table 70 Effect of processing and preparation on nutrients in cows milk

Nutrient	Concentration per 100 ml Milk			
	Before processing	After commercial evaporation and reconstitution	After dilution 1 : 1	After sterilization
Lysine (mgs)	257	195	97	74
Thiamine (mgs)	42	25	13	8
Pyridoxin (mgs)	58	29	15	7

Source: *Pediatrics*. **36**: 282, 1965.

The effects of cooking on nutrient value are virtually unpredictable. Some nutrients, like lysine, are destroyed by heat; others like ascorbic acid are destroyed when exposed to air. Food technology is very much concerned with the preservation of nutrients but no accurate figure can be offered which would represent the possible wastage of nutrients while food is processed.

Average vitamin losses based on good cooking practices are shown in Table 71.

Not all processing removes nutrients; in some instances minerals are added inadvertently and they may make an important contribution to the

Table 71 Average percentage of nutrients lost during cooking

	Thiamine	Ribo-flavin	Niacin	Ascorbic acid
Meats	35	20	25	
Meats plus drippings	25	5	10	
Eggs	25	10	0	
Cereals	10	0	10	
Legumes	20	0	0	
Vegetables, leafy green and yellow	40	25	25	60
Tomatoes	5	5	5	15
Vegetables, other	25	15	25	60
Potatoes	40	25	25	60

Source: I. C. N. N. D. Manual for Nutrition Surveys 2nd Edition, 1963.

diet. For example, the old fashioned iron cooking pot can give up its iron to the food. In Italy, tomato sauces consumed with spaghetti may contain significant amounts of iron that has been taken up in this way. A change to a more sophisticated form of living and the adoption of enamel, aluminum, or pans lined with synthetic plastic material, may mean the removal of a useful and possibly vital source of a mineral from the diet. Technology may inadvertently introduce a mineral to a diet that is naturally lacking. The introduction of metal machines for grating cassava has been shown to be responsible for the introduction of large quantities of iron into the tuber during processing (see Table 72).

Because of the variation in food composition and the influence of the many factors affecting the nutritive value of foods as consumed, it is not surprising that the assessment of diet lacks precision. The presence of inaccuracies does not mean that the use of this type of enquiry should be abandoned, for diet surveys have a definite use in the evaluation of the diets

Table 72 The iron content of untreated and of grated cassava root produced in households (mg per 100 g dry weight)

Sample	Untreated root	Grated Products	
		Made early in the day	Made later in the day
1	1.1	4.0	—
2	1.1	—	1.8
3	1.4	3.1	—
4	1.2	—	1.5
5	1.1	6.9	—
6	1.1	—	1.8
Means	1.1	4.7	1.7

Source: Hegarty, P. V. J., Wadsworth, G. R., *J. Trop. Med. and Hyg.* **71**: 51, 1968.

of groups and populations when the large sample size tends to reduce distortion of mean intakes.

It should not be assumed that the problem of assessing individual diets will be solved by the publication of food composition tables that give the nutrient values of foods *as consumed*, since it has been shown that two investigators using the same food composition tables may produce conflicting results.[30]

The discussion so far has emphasized the importance of a quantitative evaluation of diets. However, poor diet quality is as important as dietary inadequacy in the causation of protein calorie malnutrition. The unit NDpCal% has already been described (see page 220). This unit takes into account the three variable factors that determine the value of protein to the body. These factors are the quantity of protein fed, the total calorie intake, and the quality of the protein. The NDpCal% can be used to evaluate mixtures of foods. This is very necessary when diets contain protein of poor quality in low concentrations and when the total intake of food barely meets calorie requirements. The low intake may mean the protein is being burned as a source of energy, or that it is present in such low concentrations that the appetite is satisfied before protein repletion is achieved. An inadequate intake may also be due to imbalances in amino acids or antagonism between amino acids. In calculating the NDpCal% of diets a little more sophistication is added to the basic techniques described in Chapter 3.

The protein calories are calculated as before but the protein score must take into account the amino acids in all of the foods. The amount of each essential amino acid in the protein, or food, is expressed as milligrams *per gram of total essential amino acids*. This amount is then expressed as a percentage of the quantities of the same amino acid in whole egg protein (see Table 73). The lowest of these percentages is taken as the chemical score. The amino acid that is responsible for the low score is the *Limiting Amino Acid* for that particular mixture of foodstuffs. In making the calculations the sulfur amino acids, methionine and cystine, are added together. Similarly phenylalanine and tyrosine are also summed, since they are interconvertable. Examples of protein values of diets are given in Table 74.

The unit NDpCal% can also be used to evaluate whether the protein requirements of an individual are liable to be met by a diet.

Table 73   Whole egg amino acid pattern

Amino acid	A/E Ratio: mg per g of total essential amino acids	
1. Isoleucine	129	
2. Leucine	172	
3. Lysine	125	
4. Total "aromatic" amino acids:	195	
a. Phenylalanine		114
b. Tyrosine		81
5. Total sulphur-containing amino acids:	107	
a. cystine		46
b. methionine		61
6. Threonine	99	
7. Tryptophan	31	
8. Valine	141	

Source: Health Aspects of Food and Nutrition. WHO. 1969.

If an individual has a calorie requirement of 2000 and is ingesting a diet having a calorie content of 2000, then it may be stated with some degree of confidence that the requirements are being met. If however, the protein requirement is 70 grams and a diet is consumed that contains 70 grams of protein, no such conclusion can be made. The unit of weight (gram) does not describe the quality of the protein, nor does it indicate if the protein is being used for its proper purpose or energy production. The NDpCal% serves a very useful purpose in relating protein calorie requirements to protein calorie availability. The requirements for protein and calories have been specified for various ages and physiological states

Table 74 Protein values of some simplified diets. Amino acid content (mg), protein score and NDp Cal%

A. Diet I. Rice/fish/vegetable

Food Commodity (E.P.)	Grams	Calories	Protein (grams)	Calories from protein	Iso-leucine	Leucine	Lysine	Total Sulphur-containing*	Total Aromatic*	Threo-nine	Trypto-phan	Valine	Total Essential Amino Acids (E)
Rice (brown)	160	575	12.0	41	480	1,036	478	427	1,090	491	157	693	4,852
Amaranth leaves	10	5	0.46	1	22	36	23	17	43	20	7	26	194
Eggplant	30	7	0.36	1	16	22	19	6	28	13	4	18	126
Fish	40	40	7.52	30	360	578	685	304	571	344	84	460	3,386
Total	627		20.3	73	878	1,672	1,205	754	1,732	868	252	1,197	8,558
(a) A/E ratios for diet					10.2%	19.5%	14.1%	8.8%	20.2%	10.1%	2.9%	14.0%	
(b) A/E ratios for whole egg					12.9%	17.2%	12.5%	10.7%	19.5%	9.9%	3.1%	14.1%	
Percentage scores $\frac{a}{b} \times 100$					79	113	113	82	104	102	95	99	
					Limiting amino acid								

Protein score = 79

Protein calories % $= \dfrac{73}{627} \times 100 = 11.6\%$

NDpCal% = 6.0

6*

B. Diet II. Sweet potato/vegetable

Sweet potatoes 500	570	15.0	41	240	355	225	135	405	250	110	295	2,015
Amaranth leaves 50	24	2.3	6	109	179	117	85	213	98	34	128	963
Total	594	17.3	47	349	534	342	220	618	348	144	423	2,978
(a) A/E ratios for diet				11.7%	17.9%	11.5%	7.4%	20.7%	11.7%	4.8%	14.2%	
(b) A/E ratios for whole egg				12.9%	17.2%	12.5%	10.7%	19.5%	9.9%	3.1%	14.1%	
Percentage scores $\frac{a}{b} \times 100$				91	104	92	69	106	118	156	101	

Limiting amino acid

Protein score = 69

Protein calories % = $\dfrac{47}{594} \times 100 = 7.9\%$

NDpCal % = 8.0

* Sulphur-containing acids = methionine and cystine

Aromatic amino acids = Phenylalanine and tyrosine.

A = individual essential amino acid

Source: Health Aspects of Food and Nutrition. W. H. O. 1969.

for both sexes. These specifications refer to protein that is assumed to be completely utilized (*reference protein*) and having a *score* of 100.

The recommended protein and calorie requirements serve as a basis for calculating the Protein Calories Percent. For protein with a score of 100 the protein calories is the same as the NDpCal%. If, for example, the requirements for a one-year old baby are 24 grams of protein and 1200 calories, than the

$$\text{Protein Cal} = \frac{24 \times 4 \times 100}{1200} = 8$$

For reference protein the NDpCal% will also be 8.

The recommended NDpCal% at different ages and in different physiological states have been calculated and are given in Table 75. It will be seen that a diet with an NDpCal% value of less than 4.6 will not meet the needs of adult men and that a diet with an NDpCal % below 8 is incapable of meeting the needs of an infant.

Table 75 NDpCal% requirements

Age group or physiological state	NDpCal%
Birth–11 weeks	8.3
3–5 months	8.0
6–11 months	7.5
1–3 years	7.0
4–6 years	5.9
7–15 years	5.9
16 years and over (men)	4.6
16 years and over (women)	7.0
Pregnancy and lactation	9.5

The direct assessment of the nutritional status of an individual

In nutrient deprivation, the body and tissue stores are called on to make up the deficits in the diet. When the stores are depleted, the tissues themselves may be metabolized in order to maintain essential body functions. Such use is generally associated with disturbances of body function. If the deprivation continues, there will be tissue breakdown and lesions will develop that are recognized as the clinical signs of malnutrition. The sequence of events is summarized in Table 76.

As growth disturbance is probably the most important and common malfunction of the body, its measurement will be discussed first.

Table 76 The effects of malnutrition

Stage	Effect	Evaluated by
Depletion of body stores	Lowering of nutrient levels in the body stores	Biochemical levels in stores
Depletion of body tissue	Lowering of nutrient levels in tissues	Biochemical levels in tissues
	Distribution in function including growth	Physical and biophysical tests of function Anthropometry
	Anatomical lesions	Clinical signs Anthropometry
	Biochemical lesions	Changes in nutrient concentration Appearance of metabolites

Growth

Growth is a phenomenon that is associated with an increase in metabolic tissue; it is dependent on the provision of adequate nutrients. Since the growth of some tissues can be measured, anthropometry may provide a useful quantitative index of nutritional status.

Evaluation of growth requires an understanding of the patterns and ranges of normal growth, the factors causing deviations from normal growth, and an understanding of the methodology of measuring growth in the human body. Growth starts at the time of fertilization of the ovum and continues throughout intra-uterine life. After parturition, growth continues through infancy, childhood, and adolescence. Prenatal and postnatal growth are two distinct physiological periods of growth requiring separate discussion.

Prenatal Growth   From the moment of fertilization, cell multiplication takes place and at an early stage there is differentiation of cells into the three *germ* layers. The outer of these layers is the *ectoderm* from which will develop all nervous tissue, the outer layers of the skin, hair, nails, and enamel of the teeth, and some of the lining of the mouth, nose, and anal canal. The inner of the three layers is the *endoderm*; this gives rise to the entire digestive tract from the mouth to the anus, the thymus, thyroid and parathyroid glands, the trachea, lungs, liver, and pancreas. The middle layer or *mesoderm* gives rise to all of the connective tissues, bone, cartilage, blood, and the vascular system, all types of muscle, the excretory and reproductive systems, and the dermis of the skin.

Differentiation of these layers is followed by the formation of organs which are composite structures generally made up of derivatives of two of the primary germ layers. The next stage in development is the adoption of a body form; this is recognized in humans as early as the 8th week of pregnancy.

Normal gestation in humans takes place over a period of 280 days. During all of this time nutrients have to be made available to the developing fetus in order that the highly complex human organism might achieve its proper and adequate development. The rates of development for organs and tissues differ so that at any one time there must be a very special demand for nutrients, the nature of which must depend on what tissue or organ is developing, and at what rate it is growing.

Early in pregnancy the actual mass of the developing embryo is microscopical in size so that although its nutrient demands may be highly specific so far as quality is concerned, the amount required is very small. Despite the meagerness of this amount there is evidence that the dividing ovum is initially undernourished.[31] As the organism grows and develops, its physical size increases very rapidly, and the quantitative demands of the developing fetus are now very high. The scale of the increase is shown in Table 77.

Table 77   Increase in weight of the human fetus

	grams
Weight of foetus at birth	30
Weight of foetus at term	3000

Source: Widdowson, E. M., *Proc. Nutr. Soc.*, **28**: 17, 1969.

Table 78   Concentration of substances in the fetus and newborn during late pregnancy (Values are expressed as gms. per 100 gm. body wt. except for iron, which is mgm.)

Substance	Fetus 1,500 gm.	Fetus 2,500 gm.	Term infant 3,500 gm.
Protein	11.6	12.4	12.0
Fat	3.5	7.6	16.2
Water	82.5	77.3	68.8
Sodium	0.23	0.21	0.19
Calcium	0.68	0.76	0.81
Iron	7.10	7.40	7.52

Source: *Growth and Development of Children*, Fifth Edition, by E. H. Watson and G. H. Lowrey. Copyright 1967, Year Book Medical Publishers. Used by permission.

The overall rate of growth reaches a maximum at about the fourth month of gestation and then gradually decelerates for the remainder of pregnancy. Three factors, variable in magnitude and independent, determine the nutrient demands. First the rate of growth, second the increase in cell mass, and third the differentiation and development of tissues and organs at different times. Figure 91 shows diagramatically the inter-relationships of these three factors. The differentiation of the tissues has special importance towards the end of the normal gestation period when the central nervous system is developing at an extremely rapid rate (see Figure 92). The changes that take place in body composition are also considerable, again emphasizing the ever changing demand of the fetus for nutrients. Table 78 for example, shows the differential in the increase in concentration of calcium and iron as the pregnancy progresses.

The nutrition of the fetus depends on two factors; first the nutritional status of the mother, and second the placenta that is the pipeline down which the nutrients are fed. The nutrition of the mother and the fetus will now be discussed in further detail.

Nutritional status of the mother. Observations made during the Siege of Leningrad and the famine in Holland during the second World War showed

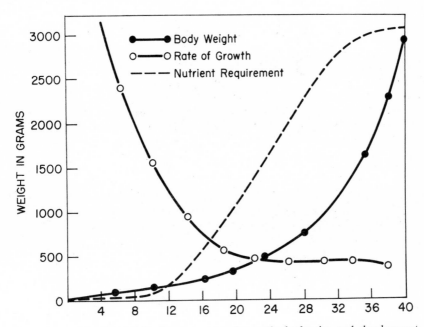

Figure 91   The relationships between rate of growth, body size and development, and nutrient requirements in the fetus

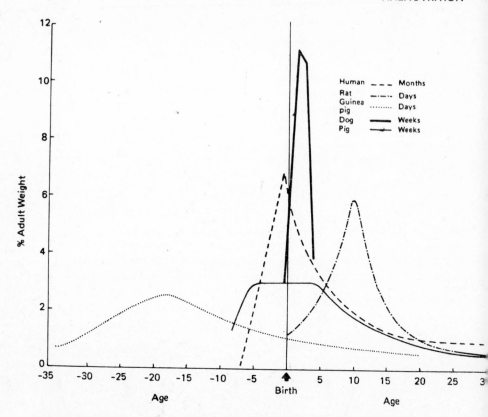

Figure 92   Rate curves of brain growth (increments in fresh weight) in relation to birth in different species. The time scale has been arbitrarily adjusted so that it is proportional to the average life span of each species (Original figure by J. Dobbing in *Applied Neurochemistry*, reproduced with the permission of Blackwell Scientific Publications Ltd., Oxford, England)

that if the mother experienced a very poor diet, conception was impossible[32,33]. If the mother conceived however, an early spontaneous termination of pregnancy was likely. The risk was especially great if the maternal malnutrition had caused some developmental abnormality.

Despite adverse conditions, pregnancy in malnourished mothers may continue for a normal gestation period, but if the fetus does not receive adequate nutrients it will be experiencing *intrauterine malnutrition* and will be born underdeveloped. There is a second possibility that the pregnancy may continue in a satisfactory way until the seventh or eighth month. The mother may then go into *premature labor* and deliver a baby that is also underdeveloped because its intrauterine life has been curtailed. If these infants have a birth weight of less than 2.5 kg they are designated as having a *low birth weight*. It is important to recognize that the low birth weight may be the product of two different sequences of events; the first being intrauterine growth retardation, and the second premature delivery. Infants of either etiology are especially at risk in the neonatal and perinatal periods of life.

Experiments with laboratory animals adds support to the observations made on humans that maternal malnutrition can give rise to abnormalities in the offspring.[34] Dogs that have been malnourished before birth remain small even when given diets of high protein value. This suggests that some irreparable damage to growth potential has taken place.[35] It has also been demonstrated that rat pups born of malnourished mothers are unable to utilize foods as efficiently as offspring born of well nourished mothers.[36] Specific nutrient deficiencies have also been incriminated as the cause of congenital abnormalities; for example vitamin A deficiency has been associated with the development of hair lips and cleft palates. A low protein diet during fetal life has been shown to affect the development of the central nervous system in animals. Deprivation is probably most serious when cell division in the brain is proceeding at a rapid rate (see Figure 92) causing a reduction of the final brain cell numbers. There is supportive evidence of this phenomenon in humans.[37]

The Pipeline After fertilization, the embryo and fetus receive nutrients in three successive ways. The initial supply is from the secretions of the "uterine glands" that feed nutrients to the free and unattached ovum during the early stages of cell division. In the second stage when a sinusoidal space is formed between the maternal and fetal tissues, nutrients pass across this layer to the developing embryo. In the final phase the nutrients are supplied through the placenta.

The food supply to the fetus usually depends on the quantity of blood reaching the fetus rather than the concentration of nutrients in the maternal plasma. This does not infer the concentration is not important; it is well known, for example, that fetal rickets can occur in the presence of maternal vitamin D deficiency. There is evidence that concentration gradients allow diffusion of nutrients across the placenta. There is also evidence of active transfer of sodium, phosphorus, iodine, and iron against the concentration gradient; this would suggest that the placenta also actively transports nutrients.

Throughout pregnancy the fetal blood level of glucose is lower than that of the mother. This is not the result of a greater consumption of glucose by the fetus but rather it is the result of the placenta maintaining a differential.

In the latter part of pregnancy glycogen storage in the liver provides an energy reserve for the new born child. If this storage is interrupted by premature delivery or is reduced by intrauterine growth failure, it can have serious implications for the infant. These have been described in Chapter 2 (see page 118).

Some lipids, such as cholesterol, are poorly transferred, while free fatty acids pass across the placenta easily in either direction.

Amino acid concentrations are usually higher on the fetal side than the maternal side of the placenta but the transfer of protein is highly selective. The function of the placenta is therefore complex and changes in its functional role may be responsible for changes in its morphology during the course of pregnancy. There is rapid placental growth in the first trimester; after this the rate of growth falls off. This phenomenon bears an inverse relationship to the increase in mass of the fetus and possibly a positive relationship to the deceleration of its growth rate.

The size of the placenta appears to be critical; smallness may be a common cause of low birth weight and not a coincidental event. Any factor which restricts the blood supply to, or from, the placenta may play an important role in the development of intrauterine malnutrition. For example, separation of the placenta late in pregnancy, and thrombosis of the placenta in diabetes may be responsible for intrauterine growth failure.

Virus infections can have a direct effect on intrauterine growth. The most commonly cited maternal infection is *Rubella*, the causative organism of *German measles*. Infection of the mother in the first trimester presents nearly a 20 per cent risk of the fetus having congenital defects; the abnormalities in growth can affect most organs and tissues. Liver and spleen enlargement, bone abnormalities, deficiencies in the clotting mechanism of the blood, heart disease, and nervous system defects have all been reported. Other viruses and microorganisms including small pox, influenza, rubeola, syphilis, and toxoplasmosis have also been incriminated as agents that interfere with intrauterine growth.

Evaluation of prenatal growth. A direct assessment of prenatal growth may be made by measurements of the new born infant. Although weight is not a true index of growth, body weight at birth can be assumed to be one measure of the gain in cell mass during intrauterine life. Low birth weight has never been attributed to a deficiency of one particular nutrient and it is widely accepted that a generally poor diet is involved.[38,39] Increases in average birth weights over a period of years have been observed in developing countries.[40] In Madrid, birth weights increased in the years following the relief of the food deprivation of the Spanish Civil War.[41]

It is possible that these increases in birth weight were due to enhanced environmental conditions, as well as improved nutritional status.

A much better index of growth achievement is obtained by measurement of body length. Measurements of infants whose gestational age is known, can be used in the preparation of growth curves. The means and standard deviations from large samples provide an expected achievement (the mean) and an upper and lower limit of normality that approximates to the third and ninety- seventh percentile. There is no standardized method of plotting curves and unfortunately the situation is confused by the availability of other curves, used by some pediatricians who define the lower limit of normality at the level of the tenth percentile.

There have been some recent efforts to produce comprehensive growth curves that describe expected achievements for several body measurements. These include body length, head, chest, trunk and limb circumference, and skinfold thickness for infants from 25 weeks to 44 weeks of age. The various measurements have also been plotted against gestational age, birthweight, and body length[42] (see Figure 93). The recording of individual measurements on such curves helps to differentiate the long, thin, malnourished baby with a large cranium who has been affected by malnutrition late in pregnancy, from the short, relatively well proportioned baby that may have been affected by the rubella syndrome early in pregnancy, or by an interruption of pregnancy.

The use of the curves is, however, not free from problems of interpretation for it is difficult to determine the exact time of conception. Frequently the last menstrual period is used as a reference point; in recent years however, the use of ovulatory inhibiting contraceptive methods has resulted in delayed ovulation. Consequently infants conceived after using "the Pill" may be some days or even a week or two younger than their calculated age and they will appear to be experiencing growth failure.

Prenatal growth curves make no differentiation between the sexes, but it is known that males are on average five per cent heavier and one per cent longer than females. This could result in the latter sex being relegated to a category of growth achievement lower than their actual achievement.

It would be advantageous if fetal size could be determined and evaluated before delivery. Precise estimates of growth can be made by x-rays but the advisability of exposing the fetus to repeated dosage of radiation is questionable. The development of ultrasonic echo sounding (sonar) promises to be a major advance in assessing fetal size in utero.[43] The principle involves the projection of intermittent or pulsed sound waves in a directional beam. The echoes are detected, and converted to an image on a cathode ray tube,

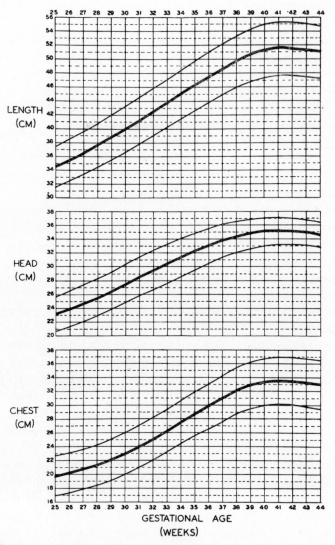

Figure 93a

Figure 93   Growth curves for new born infants. Measurements may be plotted against gestational age or birthweight (From Robert Usher and Francis Maclean: "Intrauterine growth of live born Caucasian infants at sea level: standards obtained from measurements in 7 dimensions of infants born between 25 and 44 weeks of gestation", *J. Pediat.* **74**: 901–910, 1969)

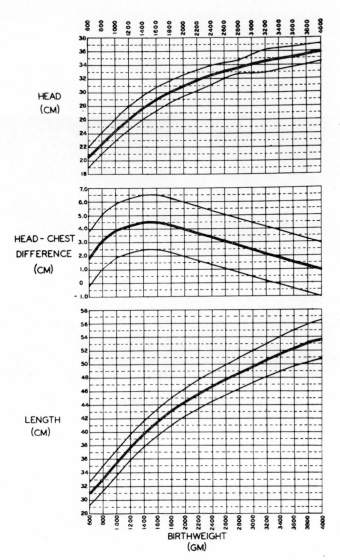

Figure 93b

and then photographed. The resultant picture (see Figure 94) provides a two-dimensional impression of the uterus and its contents. By identifying two definite points in the fetal head, it is possible to measure the distance between these points very accurately thereby enabling the measurement of the growth of the fetal head. The measurement of the developing fetus and the detection of inadequate intrauterine growth now seems feasible even before the twentieth week of life.[44]

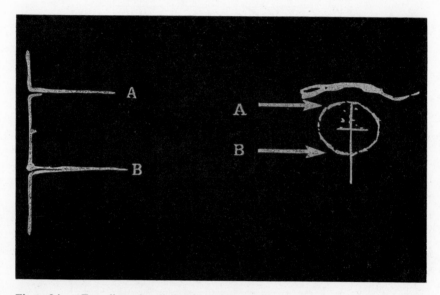

Figure 94   Two dimensional display in the transverse section of the fetal head with the ultrasonic beam bisecting it through the bi-parietal eminences exactly at right angles to the *falx cerebri*. The bi-parietal diameters are converted to vertical blips (A and B on the left) that can be measured more easily. (From Ian Donald: "Sonar as a method of studying prenatal development", *J. Pediat.* **75**: 326–333, 1969)

Post-natal growth patterns   The impetus of intrauterine growth continues after the infant is born. The velocity continues to decrease until about the fourth year of life. The child enters a middle growth period, a time of steady growth that is maintained until the twelfth year of life. The adolescent growth spurt then takes place and it is associated with a final period of several years of rapid growth (see Figure 95).

While there is a general trend, the differential in the growth of individual tissues and organs which was noted *in utero* continues and includes the rapid prenatal growth of the brain (see Figure 96). In order to accomodate the brain the cranium grows at the same time, with the result that in early

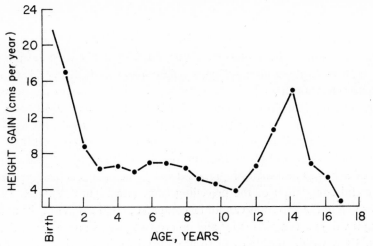

Figure 95   The pattern of incremental growth in infancy, childhood and adolescence

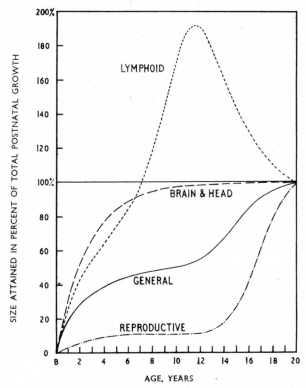

Figure 96   The differential growth of tissues. All the curves are of size attained (in per cent of the total gain from birth to maturity) and plotted so that size at age 20 is 100 on the vertical scale (From J. M. Tanner *Growth at Adolescence*, reproduced by permission of Blackwell Scientific Publications Ltd., Oxford, 1952)

life the head is quite out of proportion to the size of the body. At 12 years of age the skull of the adolescent is very often what it will be as an adult. The reproductive organs have been quiescent up to this time. They now become active and there follows a period of several years of development of the ovary, testis, and secondary sexual characteristics (see Figure 97). Other tissues grow at intermediate times, the lymphoid tissue, for example, has an active period of growth in the pre-pubescent periods of life.

There is an overall orderly fashion to growth; it starts first in the upper part of the body and then progresses distally, each stage depending on the successful completion of the preceding stage (see Figure 98).

Growth in the two sexes cannot be compared, for the onset of the adolescent growth spurt in girls is usually one to two years in advance of that of boys. Even within the sexes there are variations in the time of onset of

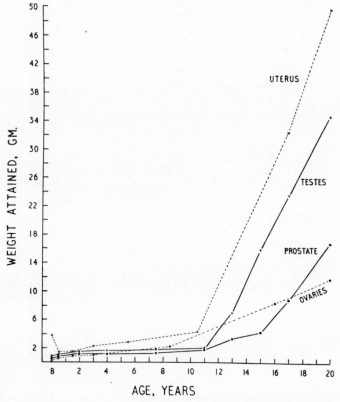

Figure 97   Growth of reproductive organs and tissues at adolescence. (From J. M. Tanner *Growth at Adolescence*, reproduced by permission of Blackwell Scientific Publications Ltd., Oxford, 1952)

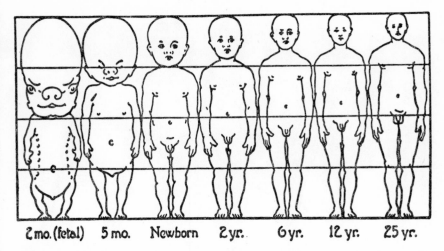

2 mo. (fetal)   5 mo.   Newborn   2 yr.   6 yr.   12 yr.   25 yr.

Figure 98   Stages of growth. The relative proportions of head, trunk and extremities for different ages. (From *Morris' Human Anatomy*, 12th edition. Copyright 1966, McGraw-Hill Book Company)

adolescence. Figure 99 shows the growth curve of several girls; at first sight it appears that they are growing at different rates. When however, they are plotted according to their time of maximum velocity, it will be seen that they have similar growth patterns and it is only the time of onset that is different.

Seasonal influences on growth have also been observed (see Figure 100). In Africa, a group of European school children living in the cool highlands had a period of maximum growth identical to that of African school children living in the hot humid coastal region at several hundred miles distance.[45]

Fat growth. Adipose tissue is found in the subcutaneous tissues where its thickness may be conveniently measured. It is also found in several other sites in the body including the perirenal area, the mesentery, and the heart. In the new born infant there is also fat of a different histological appearance which may serve like the *brown fat* of animals as an energy reserve in early life.[46]

Because subcutaneous fat is capable of being measured without too much difficulty, it is considered a valuable index of nutritional status. There have been many studies on adults which have shown a relationship between skinfold thickness and body density. Skinfold thickness is now widely accepted as a measure of adiposity. This assumption may not be true for infants and children but there is little experimental evidence to support or refute this premise. Patterns of development of skinfolds have been

7   Robson II (0314)

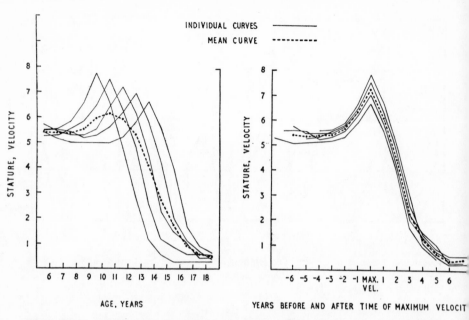

Figure 99   Relation between individual and mean velocities during the adolescent spurt. In Figure 99a, left, the height curves are plotted against chronological age; in Figure 99b, right, they are plotted according to their time of maximum velocity. (From J. M. Tanner *Growth at Adolescence* by permission of Blackwell's Scientific Publications Ltd., Oxford 1952)

described but it is not known whether these patterns follow the development of total body fat.

As in other tissues, the enlargement of adipose tissue may be due to an increase in size of the cells, an increase in numbers of cells, or a combination of both. Studies on the cellular development of adipose tissues in infants have indicated that during the first year of life there is a rapid three-fold increase in cell numbers. This is followed by a more gradual but continuous increase in numbers throughout childhood. Cell size on the other hand increases three-fold over the first six years of life. There is little change between six and thirteen years, but there is a further increase in size in adolescence.[47] This pattern of hyperplasia and hypertrophy may have considerable importance in the etiology of obesity.

Skinfold thicknesses increase from birth up to 9 months of age; there is then a decrease in thickness. This is rapid at first and it continues until the child is about 6 years of age. The fat on the trunk then increases in both boys and girls; in the limbs there is a further period of thinning in boys

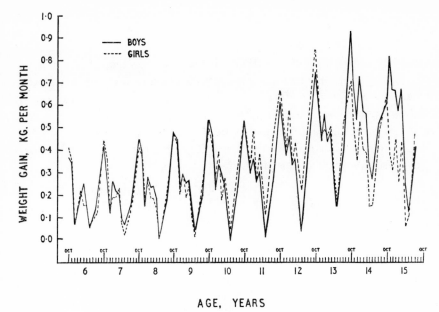

Figure 100 Seasonal patterns in growth. The annual increase in weight in both sexes between May and October is clearly seen (From J. M. Tanner *Growth in Adolescence*, reproduced by permission of Blackwell Scientific Publications Ltd., Oxford 1952)

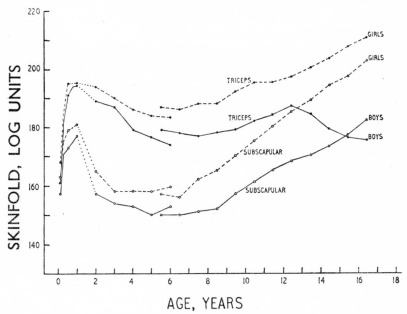

Figure 101 Development of the subscapular and upper limb fat (From J. M. Tanner *Growth at Adolescence*, reproduced by permission of Blackwell Scientific Publications Ltd., Oxford, 1952)

7*

at the time of adolescence (see Figure 101). This last phenomenon may be caused by underlying limb muscle growing more rapidly than the surrounding fat (see Figure 102). The limb is in reality a cylinder with concentric rings of muscle and fat; if the former grows more rapidly than the latter the fat will be stretched and become thinner. There is evidence that this does take place in boys, at least, for studies of the amount of DNA and RNA in muscle during growth indicates there is an active period of muscle hyperplasia from 9 years of age until growth ceases.[48]

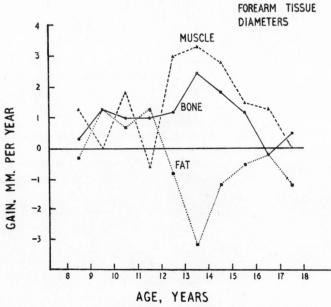

Figure 102   Changes in the diameter of the forearm tissues (From J. M. Tanner *Growth at Adolescence*, reproduced by permission of Blackwell Scientific Publications Ltd., 1952)

The growth of fat is complicated for it differs in both sexes and with age; there is also evidence that the development of fat on the trunk differs from that of the limbs. Fat may be transferred also from one site to another. While these general trends and differences are recognized, there is a real lack of specific information on the changes, therefore interpretation of measurements must be made with reservation. Because of the phenomenon of differential development, the measurement of growth in one tissue alone may be misleading. The final anthropometric evaluation means much more if height achievement is related to weight, or skinfold thickness, or other parameters of growth and development.

Factors influencing growth While growth is dependent on nutrition, it is also affected by other factors including genetic inheritance. However, although genes may contain the plan for the future growth potential of the organism, this achievement can be influenced by environmental factors including nutrition. Inheritance, environment, and nutrition, are so closely related it is impossible, except under strict controlled experimental conditions (which are impracticable so far as humans are concerned), to differentiate their respective contributions to the development of the organism. Inadequacies of growth that are observed in an individual may be due to one, or all, of these factors, and it may be impossible to decide which was responsible. From a practical point of view, it may be reasonable to assume that environmental and nutritional factors have been the main influences until such time as the genetic cause is established. The application of this assumption is far less likely to result in further deprivation of the child than assuming that an inherent brake has been applied to natural growth and development.

Genetic influences on growth The inherited influence and transmission of growth characteristics is well exemplified by the size and physique of different ethnic groups living in geographical areas of close proximity. The *Watussi* and the *Pygmies* both live in Equatorial Africa yet there is a very great difference in their average heights that undoubtedly have been determined genetically. Even where protein calorie malnutrition is widespread, tall lineages continue to produce tall children. In Central Tanzania the *Wagogo* are frequently living in famine conditions yet children still manage to achieve an adult height equivalent to their tall parents.

Differences in the height of ethnic groups may be due to genetic differences in body proportions; one group may have a long trunk and short legs, consequently the total body length may be much less than another group with the same trunk length and longer legs. The growth rates of different races may start out the same, but because of differences in the fusion of bone epiphyses, the final height of one may be much less than the other. Further evidence of the genetic influences on height is provided in studies of siblings. The relationship between the body length of sisters at birth and 17 years of age is close. When however, the lengths of a brother and sister are compared at these same ages, the relationship is much less, and is probably indicative of the control of body size by the X chromosomes. The size of offspring and parents also correlates well.

Because of genetic endowments, evaluation of growth by "normal" standards may be misleading. Figure 103 shows the growth achievement of two girls who were studied at the Fels Institute in Ohio. One was the offspring of two tall parents and the other the child of two short parents. The former is tall, and the latter is short, throughout growth. If the parental size is not taken into account it would appear that both children may be experiencing abnormal growth. This clearly indicates a need for genetically controlled growth standards.[49]

There is evidence that the proportions of fat to lean body mass may be genetically determined. Figure 104 shows the body weights of two daughters

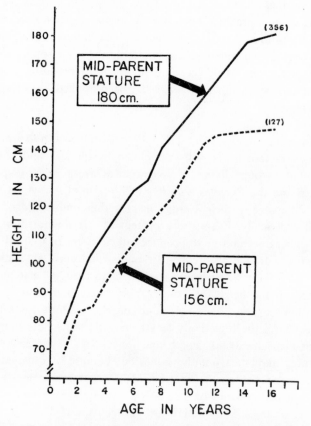

Figure 103   Effect of parental size on the statural growth of the offspring. In this example, Fels child number 356, whose midparental stature is 180 cm, markedly outpaces Fels subject number 127, whose midparental stature is 156 cm. The ultimate size difference between these two girls is in excess of 30 cm (12 inches). (Reproduced from *Interaction of Nutrition and Genetics in the Timimg of Growth* by S. M. Garn and C. G. Rohman, *Pediatric Clinics of North America* **13**, May 1966, published by W. B. Saunders Company)

born of the same mother but of different fathers. The father of one daughter had a body of averagele anness and produced a daughter of average weight. The father of the second daughter was very broad and muscular and produced a heavy daughter.

Retardation of growth caused by malnutrition does not necessarily mean that the final result of growth will be stunting. A child who has a genetic template for tallness may catch up and overtake other genetically normal individuals who may not have experienced retarded growth.

Genetically transmitted errors in metabolism may also be responsible for growth failure. In recent years there has been recognition of an increasing number of clinical conditions characterized by growth failure and which are also associated with inborn errors of metabolism.[50]

Such syndromes are relatively rare however, compared with growth failure associated with environmental and nutritional inadequacies.

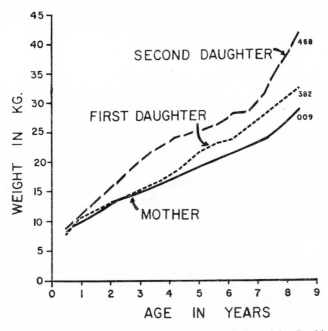

Figure 104   Effect of parental body size on the growth in weight. In this example, involving the same mother and 2 different husbands, the growth and weight of the children markedly reflect the lean body mass of their fathers. Child number 468 has a father with a lean body mass of approximately 80 kg, while her half-sibling number 382 represents a parental lean body mass of approximately 60 kg. (Reproduced from *Interaction of Nutrition and Genetics in the Timing of Growth* by S. M. Garn and C. G. Rohman, *Pediatric Clinics of North America*, **13**, May 1966, published by W. B. Saunders Company)

Nutritional and environmental influences on growth The effects of repeated minor illness are not easy to evaluate because body measurement
is difficult, and errors in measuring length over short periods of time may
be large compared with the growth increment. When measurements are
only taken at wide intervals of time the catch-up process may mask the
deficit in growth. If children suffer severe or prolonged illness, then the
effects on growth become more obvious. It is often difficult to blame the
growth failure on illness alone, because children who become seriously ill
are frequently from families lacking skilled maternal care and regular
nutritious meals.

It has been claimed that exercise will accelerate growth but it is virtually
impossible to design an adequately controlled experiment that will allow
comparisons of the effects of energy expenditure on growth. Consequently,
no definite conclusions have been made on this subject.

Socio-economic class Marked differences have been observed in the
heights and weights of different socio-economic classes (see Figure 105).
The growth of children in the highest social class representing professional
persons, employers, and salaried staff is more advanced than the manual
wage earners. The causes are probably multiple and include nutrition,
home conditions, poor environmental hygiene, and increased risks of infection. There may also be a relationship to the height of the parents. It has
been observed in Scotland that the short women take less skilled jobs and
marry short men who also tend to have less skilled occupations. The investigators believed that height appeared to favor socio-economic advance-
ment so that larger people have a greater capacity to rise in the social
scale, while the shorter individuals remain in the lower socio-economic
groups.[51] This might not be a direct cause and effect relationship.

Family size The size of the family also exerts an effect on growth.
Even within the higher socio-economic classes, the mean height of children
in families with four or more children is significantly less than the mean
height of children with less than four children (see Figure 105). This may
be the result of competition for food, or lack of individual attention.

The secular trend Over the last century there has been a speeding up
of growth processes (see Figure 106) in the same ethnic groups, living in
the same, or even different geographical location. For example, the English
schoolboys at Marlborough College, aged 16.5 years, had an average height
of 65.5 inches in 1873. In 1953, they averaged 69.6 inches in height. This
represents a gain of 4.1 inches in 70 years or one-half inch every decade.[52]
Similarly Japanese children living in the United States are taller than their
ethnic compatriots in Japan.[53]

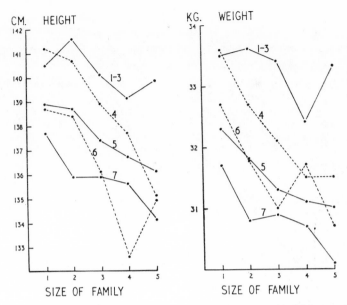

Figure 105   Relation between height and weight of 11 year-old children and size of family in different socio-economic classes. Classes 1–3 represent professional persons, employers and salaried staff. Class 4 is made up of non-manual wage earners, Class 7 represents unskilled manual wage earners (From *Growth at Adolescence* by J. M. Tanner, reproduced by permission of Blackwell Scientific Publications Ltd., Oxford, 1952)

Malnutrition, infection, and nutrient deficiency   Growth failure is the one constant feature of protein calorie malnutrition. Interference with growth is a commonplace phenomenon that is observed in children who have been subject to repeated or prolonged infections. It is not surprising therefore to find that economically depressed communities, or those having an environment favoring communicable disease transmission, have children with growth performances below that of other better endowed populations. However the presence of a high incidence of an infective agent (*Schistosomiasis*) does not necessarily mean additional growth retardation.[54] Specific nutrient deficiencies can also lead to growth failure. For example, in rickets there is a disturbance in bone growth that is reflected in height deficits. In chronic malnutrition and undernutrition the growth of epiphyses may be inhibited over a period of years; when fusion eventually takes place it will result in a permanently stunted child. Iodine and zinc deficiency is also associated with stunting of growth. Other causes of stunting of growth, that are not primarily nutritional in origin, are very numerous and beyond the scope of this book.[55]

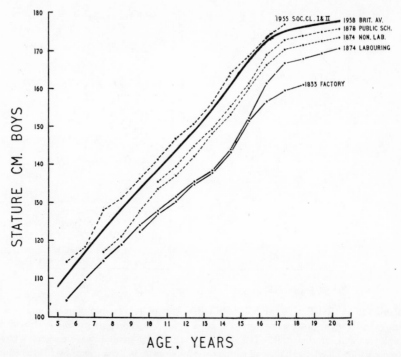

Figure 106   Height of English boys 1833–1958 to show secular trend. 1833 factory boys, 1874 laboring and non-laboring classes, 1878 'public' school (upper classes), 1955 social class 1 and 2, 1958 British average. (From *Growth at Adolescence* by J. M. Tanner, reproduced by permission of Blackwell Scientific Publications Ltd., Oxford, 1952)

Failure to Thrive   In recent years increasing attention has been given to a clinical syndrome known by a variety of names such as "Failure to Thrive", "Environmental Retardation",[56] "Hospitalism"[57], "Affect Deprivation"[58], "Emotional Deprivation"[59], and "Dwarfism"[60]. The commonest cause of this now well recognized pediatric problem has been stated to be short parents; in actual fact the true nature and extent of this condition is not clear. The syndrome was originally observed in children and infants exposed to prolonged periods of emotional deprivation in institutions and hospitals. The observations of Widdowson on the growth of children in two orphanages in Germany clearly showed the adverse effects of a poor emotional environment on growth[61] (see Figure 107). The diet and availability of food in both orphanages were the same, but in one the average weight gain of children was about one-third of the other. The group with adequate weight gain was given supplementary bread but over the next 6-month period of observation, the mean weight gain was less than it had been before supplementation. There was a sharp increase in mean weight during the same period in the other orphanage where the weight gain previously had been slow. Some factor was obviously counteracting the beneficial effect of the supplementary food; this was eventually traced to the overbearing and critical attitude of the supervisor of one of the orphanages.

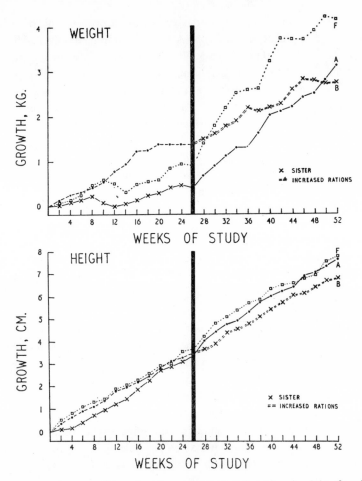

Figure 107   Influence of sister-in-charge on growth in height and weight of orphanage children. The presence of the sister is marked by X plots, increased rations by = —. Orphanage B diet supplemented at time indicated by the vertical bar but the sister was simultaneously transferred from A (—) to B (- - -). The magnitude of growth follows the presence or absence of the sister not the amount of the rations. The curves F represents favorites of the sister transferred with her from B to A. (Original data of Widdowson, Lancet 1: 1316, 1951. Figure from *Growth at Adolescence* by J. M. Tanner, reproduced by permission of Blackwell Scientific Publications Ltd., Oxford 1952)

As *failure to thrive* is becoming more widely recognized as a disease entity, cases are now being observed in families.[62] Although the criteria for this disease are neither clear-cut, nor firmly established, it has been suggested that children who have not achieved the third percentile for height and weight on accepted growth standards should be suspected as infants and children who are *failing to thrive*.[63,64]

The syndrome may include overt signs of malnutrition, and retardation of motor and social development.[65] Affected children may have abnormal feeding patterns and many have feeding difficulties.[66] In most cases there are no clinical or laboratory findings to account for the disruption of growth. The majority of cases are under two years of age and many are born with a weight deficit at birth. Family disruption, parental immaturity, large family size, and postpartum mental depression, have been associated with its development, although these problems may not be present consistently. The threat to health of *failure to thrive* is not fully understood, but retarded growth and mental retardation in older children may represent the residual effects of this syndrome.

Diagnosis is usually based on clinical histories, pediatric, psychiatric and psychological testing, and selective investigations to exclude hormonal imbalances, and inborn errors of metabolism. Cases normally respond to treatment which includes the provision of adequate emotional stimulation. Patients are usually discharged for further surveillance by social service departments.

No matter how efficient the diagnostic services and treatment may be, it would seem essential to detect these cases at an early stage and reduce the risk of possible physical or developmental retardation. The *iceberg analogy* of protein calorie malnutrition also applies to *failure to thrive* (see page 30). The children seen in clinics and hospitals may represent the "clinically apparent" cases above the surface of the water. A vast number of "clinically inapparent" cases may be submerged in the community and they may remain unrecognized until diagnostic and screening tools are improved, and applied in the community. It may be possible by increasing surveillance over the infant and growing child, to detect these cases in the early stages of the disease. By using sociological techniques, it also may be possible to detect families at risk. Through the provision of direct aid or appropriate services, home and family break-up may be avoided thereby preventing further deterioration in the situation.

Failure to thrive is an expression of the negative influences of the environment on growth. The positive effects of the environment in countering growth retardation have also been reported. Significant differences in height between Puerto Ricans born in New York and Puerto Rico have been noted, and it was found that the longer the residence in New York the better the growth performance of the children.[67] It appears that the inherent drive for growth achievement that had been inhibited in Puerto Rico was stimulated by living conditions in New York City. Whether the inhibiting factors in Puerto Rico were diet or infection cannot be established but there can be little doubt about the beneficial effects of a more favorable environment on growth.

Maturity   Puberty is a period when the growth rate accelerates and the individual starts to achieve sexual maturity. For these reasons, it is a time of considerable anxiety for parents and the adolescent. It is therefore important to recognize the various factors which influence maturity and its onset.

Genetic influence   The timing of sexual maturation, like growth, is under genetic control. Puberty is associated with a considerable increase in body size. It therefore follows that body size at any time in puberty is not only controlled by the genetic influences on growth, but also by the genetic influences that decide whether the child will be early or late in maturing. A child that is genetically a "late starter" will have an apparent deficit in growth compared with children of the same age or with children having a more advanced onset of maturity. It has already been shown that the actual growth that takes place may be identical in magnitude to that of other children (see Figure 99, page 410).

Environmental influences   Studies performed in many regions of the world have shown that an accelerated onset of menarche associated with acceleration of physical growth, follows a major improvement in socio-economic conditions. Socio-economic factors also influence nutrition, public and individual health, and family size. Because of the inter-relationships between these factors, an evaluation of the individual components is impossible.

The age of onset of menarche differs markedly by social class. In Bavaria, high social class and adequate nutrition are associated with an earlier onset of menarche.

In the United States, menarche has been observed to occur earlier in southern-born and northern-born Negroes reared in the North than girls reared in the South. Within income groups it has been noted that both Whites and Negroes had similar ages of onset of menarche. Within the total population the lower age of onset was associated with the economically privileged.[68]

Table 79 The influence of social class on
onset of menarche

Social class	Mean age of onset years
Upper	12.9
Middle	14.4
Peasants	16.4

Source: Stratz, C. H., *Der Körper des Kindes und seine Pflege*, (9th. Ed., Stuttgart Ferdinand Enke, 1922).

In South Africa, it has been observed that Bantu girls in the more southern temperate climates had better physiques, less evidence of malnutrition or specific disease, and earlier menarche than those living in hotter northern areas where bilharzia, malaria, and malnutrition were prevalent.[69]

In other studies, diets have been classified according to their nutrient value and it has been noted that diets rich in protein are associated with earlier onset of menarche.[70] Conversely, nutritional deprivation during the second World War was associated with delays in menarche.[71]

In low income families, the age of menarche has been delayed in families with many siblings[72] but it is accelerated by migration from a rural to an urban environment.[73]

Evaluation of growth

The evaluation of growth depends on two factors, the practical limitations of physical measurements and the range of normality.

A description of the methodology of body measurement is beyond the scope of this book and the reader is referred to standard references on this subject.[74,75]

Weight This is a summation of fat, body water, and the lean cell mass and it is not a true index of the amount of metabolic tissue present in the body. Changes in weight may be due to loss or gain of fat, fluid, or metabolic tissue, so that care is required in interpreting weight data.

Frequently the measurement of weight is inaccurate. Errors may be due to faults in the design of the scales, inadequate training of personnel, and inaccurate recording of data. While a skilled observer should be able to weigh within 100 grams of the true weight, observations on the accuracy of weighing methods in a baby clinic have revealed errors as large 2.5 kg.[76] Even though the weighing machines may be accurate and used by a skilled operator, there may be seasonal discrepancies in weights if the subject is weighed in heavy clothes in the winter and light clothes in the summer.

Fat Subcutaneous fat can be measured easily by means of skinfold calipers. These instruments pinch a double thickness of skin and the intervening fat between two plates having a standard contact area and exerting a constant pressure. The *Harpenden and Lange calipers* are the two most commonly used. In the hands of trained observers these instruments are capable of obtaining accurate, reproducible measurements of skinfold (fat) thickness. Measurements are made at several sites. Usually these are over the back of the arm (*triceps*), the *subscapular* region, the *abdomen*, and the *suprailiac* region. It has been suggested that measurements from these sites can be used to estimate total body fat and the quantity of the calorie reserves.[77,78,79]

Skinfolds are also being used as a measure of leanness and obesity.[80] There is evidence, however, that there are ethnic differences in the distribution of fat throughout the body,[81,82] in which case it is unacceptable to pool data gathered from different ethnic groups.

Linear measurements

Two types of linear measurement are used. The first evaluates body height or length, and the second measures the circumference of the head, chest, or limbs. When measuring body length, the young infant is placed in a reclining position. Later, when it is able to stand, height is measured upright. Measurements of reclining body length should not be compared with those of height because even in the same person there is a discrepancy in measurements taken by both methods caused by some sagging of the trunk, and bowing of the spinal column in the upright position.

Total body length or height represents the sum of the length of the legs, the trunk, and the skull. When there are ethnic differences in body proportion, it may be necessary to measure each of these components separately to see if one of them is making a particular contribution to height. The circumference of the head is used as an indirect measurement of brain size.[83,84] The circumference of the chest and the head are approximately the same for the first six months of life, but after this the chest circumference increases at a more rapid rate than the head. Between the ages of six months and five years of age, a chest to head ratio of less than unity may be indicative of a failure to develop, or to wasting of the muscle and fat of the chest wall. It may therefore be a useful ratio for evaluating protein calorie malnutrition.

Examination of the transverse section of the arm shows that it represents three concentric sleeves, the inner bone, the middle muscle mass and an outer sleeve of skin and subcutaneous fat. If the circumference of the arm is known, it is possible to calculate the circumference of the muscle (see Figure 108). Measurements made midway between the shoulder and the elbow provide a mid-arm muscle circumference. It is usually assumed that this measurement is giving a true indication of muscle volume and that the diameter of the bone is constant in size. Although there is no justification for this assumption, the mid-arm muscle circumference nevertheless correlates well with protein calorie adequacy.[85]

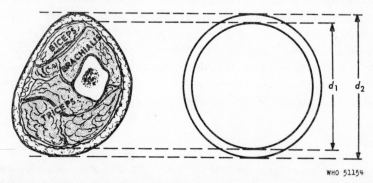

WHO 51154

Figure 108   Calculation of mid-upper-arm-muscle-circumference. Measurements are made of the arm circumference C_2 and triceps skinfold S. Let $d_1 =$ muscle diameter and $d_2 =$ arm diameter then skinfold $S = 2x$ subcutaneous fat $= d_2 - d_1$ and the arm circumference $= \pi d_2$.

Now the muscle circumference $C_1 = \pi d_1 = \pi[d_2 - (d_2 - d_1)]$
$$= \pi d_2 - \pi(d_2 - d_1)$$

Hence $C_1 = C_2 - \pi S$. (From *Assessment of Nutritional Status of the Community* by D. B. Jelliffe, WHO. Monograph No. 53, 1966)

Standard values are available but these do not take into account ethnic differences in fat thickness over the triceps region which may invalidate their use.

A more accurate measurement of soft tissue thickness may be obtained from radiographs; these can differentiate the skin and subcutaneous fat, and muscle and bone. Radiographs of the chest may also be used to evaluate soft tissue thickness in the first five years of life.[86]

Linear measurements are influenced by genetic factors, nutritional status, and the variability in patterns of maturing. The variability removes much of the meaning of chronological age. This is especially true in adolescence, when an achievement in years of life may bear no close relationship to the progress that has been made towards achieving adulthood. Because of the difficulties of relating growth to age, radiographs of bones are being used to evaluate growth achievement over a period of time. It is well known that skeletal development is slowed in malnutrition; consequently, the timing of fusion of the epiphyses of growing bones can be used as an index of the amount of delay in growth at a given time. Observation on well nourished populations have established standards for fusion of various bone epiphyses, and radiographs of subjects may be compared with the standard. It is not uncommon for skeletal growth of malnourished children to be 30 per cent behind that expected for a given chronological age. Ossification of the bony centers of the hand and wrist are reliable measures of skeletal development, and radiographs of the hand and wrist can be used to evaluate growth retardation right up to, and beyond, menarche.[87,88]

Normal growth

Any measurement of growth is the product of a "built-in" genetic target which has been influenced by nutritional and environmental factors. In practice the identification of the contribution of each component is not as important as making the decision on whether the measurements lie within the limits of normality.

Because there is a wide variation in patterns of growth, averages of individual measurements are not helpful in defining normality for the whole body. It is unlikely that a person will succeed in achieving an average height *and* an average weight *and* an average arm circumference *and* an average skinfold thickness at several sites all at the same time. It is necessary therefore, to describe a range of measurements that encompass normality, and how far a particular measurement deviates from that normal range. The limits of normality are arbitrary and their extent will depend on the purpose for which the data are to be used.

The range of normality for selecting well-muscled adolescents for training in wrestling will for example, be much more limited than the range used for general purposes of screening school children. For the latter, it is usual to define as abnormal those children whose measurements are found in only the upper and lower three per cent of a similar population of healthy individuals (the 3rd and 97th percentiles).

In order to define the limits of normality in healthy populations, large numbers of children are measured at particular ages. From this data a smooth curve can be prepared that absorbs individual variations. Standard curves obtained in this way are however, only representative of the sample which provided the data. From the description of the varying influences on growth, it is apparent that standards may not be widely applicable.

It is obvious that there must be separate standards for the two sexes, and it is equally apparent that standards for children in the United States should not be applied, for example, to the children of New Guinea. It may be argued further that the use of standards developed for one geographical location and used for the evaluation of groups from other parts of the same country, has questionable validity. However, one national standard has the advantage that it may draw attention to an area where growth appears to be unsatisfactory, thereby stimulating further inquiry to see if the problem has nutritional origins. Until more appropriate data become available existing standards will have to be used, but their limitations should be recognized.

Data are usually collected in surveys of the cross-sectional type. Measurements collected on this one occasion are then used as an index of achievement at a particular point in time. Even if adequate and appropriate standards are available, this single measurement tells little of the dynamics of indi-

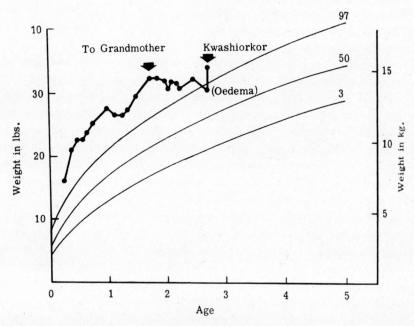

Figure 109   Weight record of Child *A* suffering from kwashiorkor. This boy had a satisfactory weight until his second birthday, when for social reasons he went on a poor diet and 9 months later developed kwashiorkor. A single measurement at the end of this period would give little indication of the deterioration in his growth performance. (Reproduced from *Transactions of the Royal Society of Tropical Medicine and Hygiene*, **62:** 200, 1968, with the permission of Dr. David Morley)

vidual growth. When the measurements are compared with normal standards, they may appear to be satisfactory or unsatisfactory. However, it is quite possible that the child who appears to have achieved good growth may be experiencing growth failure, while the child who has an apparent unsatisfactory performance may be growing at an exceptionally good rate. Figures 109 and 110 illustrate two such cases. Child A was an exceptional child having a growth velocity in excess of the 97th percentile. There was a breakdown in the family and the boy was sent to live with his grandmother who failed to feed him adequately. If the last measurement had been the only one available, the observer would have been misled. The previous record clearly shows how a satisfactory growth performance had deteriorated to an existing unsatisfactory level. Child B has suffered from nutritional deprivation but is gaining weight rapidly. Although he has not yet reached the third percentile and his achievement is still unsatisfactory, he is nevertheless experiencing a satisfactory period of catch-up growth. These two cases illustrate the value of repeated measurements taken over a period of time. This procedure not only allows comparisons to be made with normal standards at various points in time, but even more important, it is possible to observe changes in growth velocity in the individual. Longitudinal growth studies are not feasible in nutritional surveys, but they should be one of its by-products. If the practice of measuring children throughout life can be encouraged, the accumulation of data may be used eventually for the development and establishment of growth standards that take into account the ethnic composition of the community, geographical location, socio-economic strata, and secular trends.

Growth velocities can be computed from repeated measurements and used to evaluate incremental growth. It has been pointed out already that growth is not a steady affair. The velocity of growth decelerates from birth onwards and for some years there is a plateau which is succeeded by the adolescent growth spurt. If serial measurements are available, recent growth velocity may be compared with past performance. If velocity standards are available, then an individual velocity may be compared with the standard throughout the growing period. The methodology of measuring children in clinics is probably satisfactory but the lack of subsequent use of the data makes it virtually worthless. If no chart is available for plotting the data, the weight or height should be noted in the record of each individual child. All too often the data are recorded in books or even on loose sheets of paper and may never be related to the health or nutritional status of the child. The practice of recording growth data in a proper fashion is important and deserves further detailed discussion.

8*

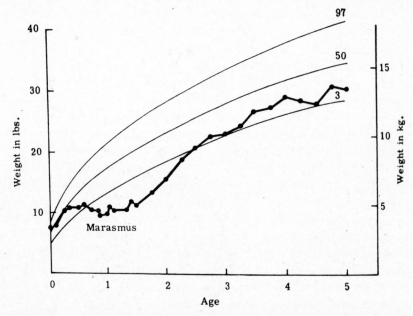

Figure 110   Weight record of child *B* recovering from maramus. This child at the age of five years is experiencing a satisfactory period of *catch-up* growth. A single measurement would indicate a poor growth achievement and would give no indication of the *catch-up* phenomenon (Reproduced from *Transactions of the Royal Society of Tropical Medicine and Hygiene*, **62**: 200, 1968 with the permission of Dr. David Morley)

Recording of growth

Growth Charts   There are several kinds of growth charts. They may give graphic plots of weight or height by age, or height for weight, head circumference by age, weight velocity by age, or height velocity by age.

Weight by Age   These are being used increasingly in many countries that are developing standards appropriate to local conditions. They are often used to detect early malnutrition by evaluation of weight.[89,90,91] It is the practice in many countries for the mother to keep the record. This probably helps to arouse and maintain interest in growth and enables the mother and father to observe the progress in weight gain within the "paths of normality" over a period of several years (see Figure 111).

Height and Weight by Age   In industrialized countries combined height and weight charts are in common use (see Figure 112). Unfortunately the data used to prepare some of these charts are 30–40 years old and, because of the secular trends, the standards may be too low for well nourished populations. Recently height and weight curves at decimal ages for English

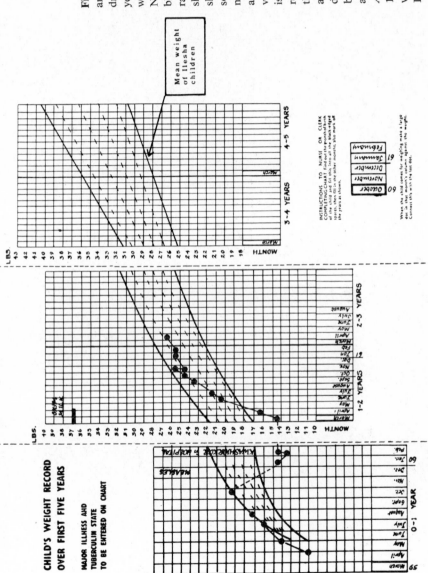

Figure 111 A health and weight chart for children from birth to five years of age. This chart was developed for use in Nigeria. The continuous black lines indicate the range in which the weight should fall. The chart shows the weight loss associated with an attack of measles and kwashiorkor, and the subsequent recovery of weight. The chart is also used as a health record, and record of the child's immunization against communicable disease. (Original figure by W.J.F. Cutherbertson and D. Morley, in *West African Medical Journal*, **11**:237, 1962, reproduced with permission of Glaxo Laboratories Ltd.)

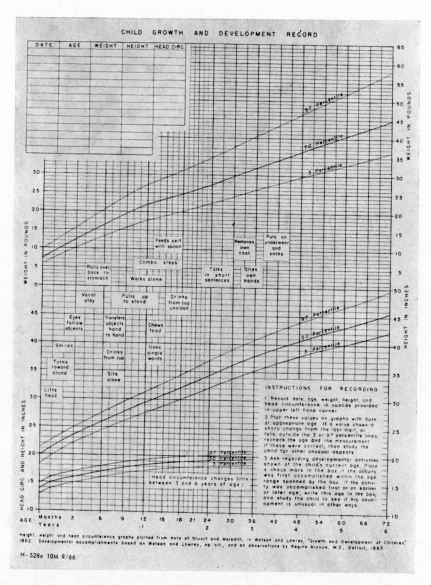

Figure 112   The child growth and development record. This is typical of charts used in health agencies in the United States (Reproduced with permission of the Michigan State Department of Public Health)

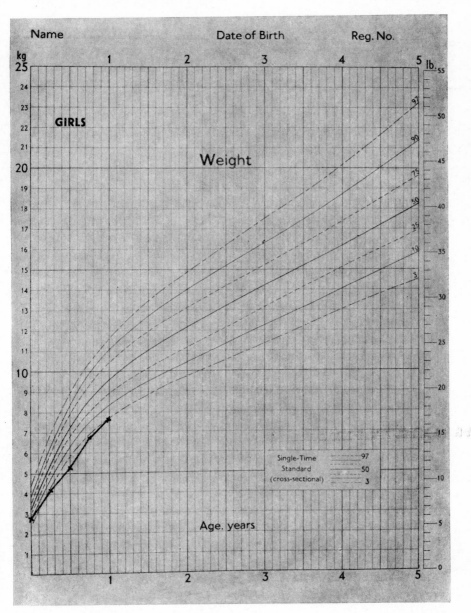

Figure 113   Weight chart of a small female child. During the first year of life she appears to be growing at the rate of a child in the third percentile (Weight chart reproduced with permission of Dr. J. M. Tanner)

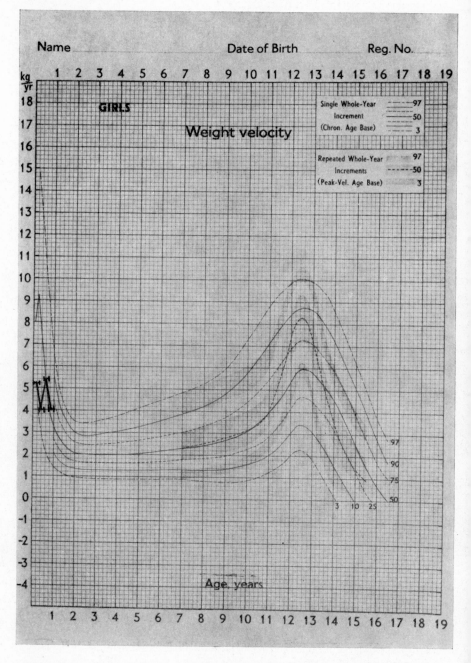

Figure 114   Weight velocity chart of the same child. This shows that the child has experienced *less deceleration* of growth than a child in the fiftieth percentile. (Velocity chart reproduced with permission of Dr. J. M. Tanner)

school children have been published.[92] These are available from birth to five years, and from birth to 18 years. Velocity curves have also been prepared for height and weight, from birth to 18 years, and are also based on decimal age. The graphic recording of velocity gives a greater insight into growth patterns than the traditional plotting of height or weight achievement. Figure 113 shows the weight of a female child during her first 12 months of life; according to her record, weight gain follows the third percentile. When the velocity (see Figure 114) of growth is calculated by three-month periods and plotted on velocity curves, the evaluation changes. Between birth and three months the deceleration of velocity of weight gain was greater than expectations, but since that time, the velocity of weight gain was greater than that for children in the fiftieth percentile.

Physique charts In large samples of the population, it is possible to establish mean values which represent average height and average weight. Children whose measurements comply both for height and weight with these mean values may be considered as having a "Normal Physique" for that population. When averages for height and weight are known at different ages it is possible to plot a curve representing mean height and weight by age.[93] The height and weight of an individual can be plotted on these charts and compared with the standard.

Figure 115 shows a physique chart prepared from measurements of London school boys. It will be seen that Child A is underweight for his height although his height compares favorably for the "normal" standard for that age. Child B is overweight for his height; he is also overweight and underheight by "normal" standards. Child C is underweight and underheight for his age, but his weight is normal for his height. This boy appears to have a normal physique but his achievement is only that of a younger child. He may be retarded in growth, or he may be genetically small; a point which may be clarified by measuring the height of the parents.

When using physique charts it is not necessary to know the age of the child; this is a great advantage in many developing countries where the date of birth may not be known. The child may be "fitted" into a physique group that resembles his own; continued observation will show whether he is maintaining pace with his peers or whether his physique is changing. Figure 116 is the record of an African schoolboy who was persistently underweight for his height. During the course of regular weighing sessions, the school teacher noted that he appeared to be overweight. As his physical appearance belied this, he was referred for medical examination. It was found that he had edema, severe anemia, and intestinal parasites. During antihelminthic treatment, more than a pound of roundworms were evacu-

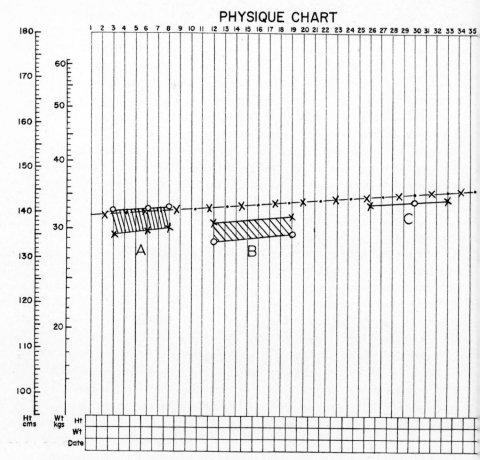

Figure 115   Physique Chart. The line *x---x---x* is the standard for that community, and is the line that should be followed by school boys over a three year period. Child A is underweight for his height which is above 'normal'. Child B is overweight for his height which is below 'normal'. Child C has a normal physique

ated. The weight gain caused by the accumulation of fluid, and the worms, might not have been noticed on a cursory examination of the child. There is little doubt that physique graphs can play a useful role in evaluating health and nutritional status. They also have the advantage that local standards can be prepared easily.

The physique chart may include a curve that represents the borderline of malnutrition. This is particularly useful in community survey work (see Figure 117) when the data may be plotted on a chart and used for comparative purposes.[94]

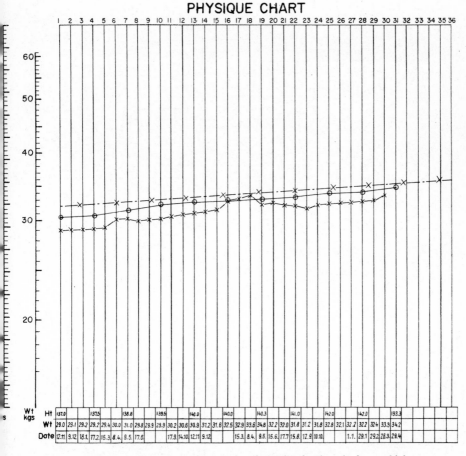

Figure 116 Physique chart of an African schoolboy who developed edema which was first detected in the regular weighing sessions of the class

A *Malnutrition score* can be calculated. This is a useful method of evaluating nutritional status and the effects of public health programs on communities. The first step in this calculation is the establishment of a minimum standard weight curve (*The malnutrition line*) which should be surpassed by children. It has been suggested that two-thirds of the mean weight for age of well nourished children in the community should be used as a standard.[95] The percentage of children below the *malnutrition line* is the *malnutrition score* and it can be calculated periodically. It should be noted that all children falling below the minimum standard for weight are not necessarily malnourished, nor does it mean that all children above the standard are

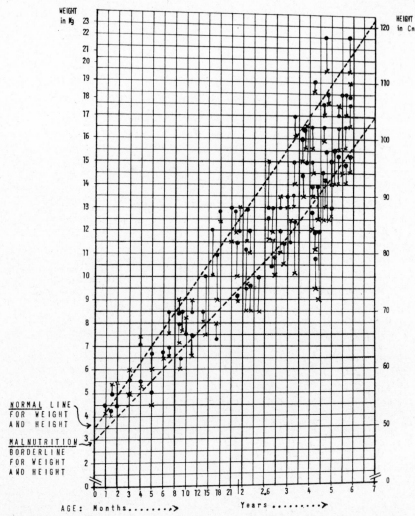

Figure 117   Weight and height chart from a community survey. The use of such a chart assists in the appraisal of the growth achievement of the community (Reproduced from *Health Aspects of Food and Nutrition* WHO Western Pacific Regional Office Manila 1969)

well nourished. Although the *Malnutrition score* is not a direct index of nutritional status it has considerable practical value in evaluation of nutrition projects.

Clinical evaluation

Clinical signs appear relatively late in the cycle of events of malnutrition (see Table 76, page 397). In some circumstances the signs of malnutrition can be quite distinctive and unmistakable; for example, the *Casals necklace* of pellagra (see page 37 and plate 7). Unfortunately most of the signs of malnutrition are not so distinctive. The value of clinical signs depends on their specificity. This means that they should always be present when a particular nutrient is deficient and they should not occur in other non-nutritional disease states. Angular stomatitis (see plate 9) associated with riboflavin deficiency is not specific since it is also seen in pellagra. Clinical signs should also be sensitive, which infers that few cases should lack the sign. A full description of signs associated with malnutrition is beyond the scope of this book and readers seeking further information should refer to standard works on this subject.[96,97,98]

Eleven clinical signs have been listed as suggestive of protein calorie malnutrition: edema, dyspigmentation of the hair, pluckability of hair, thin sparse hair, straight hair, muscle wasting, depigmentation of the skin, psychomotor change, moon face, hepatomegaly, and flaky paint dermatosis.

Few of these signs are specific to protein calorie malnutrition, nor are they all sensitive. In addition to this, the signs are subjective and difficult to standardize. Their interpretation is further complicated by their varying patterns in the different areas of the world where protein calorie malnutrition is prevalent. The character of skin rashes is affected by other nutrient deficiencies and by secondary infections with micro-organisms.

Clinical signs are a feature of several other nutrient deficiency diseases which have been induced experimentally; however deficiency of a single nutrient is most unlikely to occur in real life. Because deficiencies are usually multiple, clinical signs may differ widely from the classical descriptions of text books. To complicate the picture still further, atypical lesions or signs may appear early in the course of the disease and malnutrition may not be suspected because other indications of nutritional inadequacy are absent.

The ambiguities and difficulties can be minimized to some extent by training personnel in the recognition of signs of malnutrition. Before nutrition surveys are undertaken it is important to insure that definitions of signs are standardized, and that the criteria for stating whether a sign is present are fully understood by the observers. Colored slides, plates, films, and patients suffering from deficiency disease, may be used to achieve uniformity of reporting.

During the course of a clinical evaluation it is customary for the state of the teeth and gums to be noted. Mottling of the teeth is usually considered diagnostic of fluorosis. It can occur also in other conditions.

The presence of decayed, missing or filled teeth (DMF) is often used to record *caries* in a community. There is a probable relationship between the intake of carbohydrate foods (particularly those that contain sugars and are sticky) and dental caries, but the DMF record is not an index of nutritional status. Teeth may be affected by gum disorders which have a nutritional etiology, but there are other conditions of the gums that are unrelated to food or nutrition, and these may also be the cause of missing teeth.

Biochemical assessment of nutritional status

In nutrient deprivation, the depletion of nutrients may be reflected in lower nutrient levels in the stores and the tissues. In certain circumstances these may be measured. As the deprivation state continues the tissue damage and disturbances in function may be accompanied by biochemical lesions. These are characterized by the appearance of metabolites or changes in enzyme levels.

In the laboratory where experimental conditions can be controlled, biochemical determinations play an important role in the evaluation of nutritional status. In life, the situation is far more complex and the value of biochemical tests as indices of nutritional status is currently under critical review by many scientists. Interrelationships between nutrients and the multiple nature of deficiencies in real life, complicate and cloud the biochemical picture. Depletion of several nutrients may be taking place at different rates and the body may be making attempts to adapt its function to these deficiencies.

The biochemical response also depends on the relative proportions of protein and calories in the diet and even the source of the calories.[99] If the intake of calories is inadequate for energy needs, the diversion of protein as an energy source may deprive the body of essential amino acids required for enzyme systems.

If the deficiency is caused by poor quality protein, the metabolic changes in the body depend on the amino acid pattern of the protein in the diet. One particular pattern may allow the synthesis of some enzymes but not others.

Secondary deficiencies can also arise because a deficiency of one nutrient may lead to disturbances in the metabolism of another. For example, vitamin A deficiency frequently complicates protein calorie malnutrition. Vitamin A may be essential for the structural integrity of some of the cell organelles and consequently cell function. It is possible that protein metabolism may be affected if the function of the organelles is disturbed. Conversely, protein deficiency may prevent the removal of vitamin A from the liver so that tissue deficiency may be occurring before the stores of vitamin A are depleted. Infections and infestations, common in malnourished populations, also influence the biochemical patterns of amino acids in the blood.[100]

The choice of the biochemical test will depend on several factors, the first of which is the objective of the test. If the test is to be used for research purposes it should be highly specific; if it is to be used for clinical screening then less fine measurement is required. Secondly, consideration has to be given to the specimen and whether it is easily collected, stored, and transported. Blood is sometimes very difficult to collect; urine demands special storage and transport facilities in hot climates, or in remote areas. Thirdly, ability to use a complex test will depend on the availability of skilled manpower to collect the specimen and complete the laboratory procedure; this latter is of course related to the facilities and resources of the laboratory.

Interpretation of Data   This presents many problems. Ideally, the test should reflect the nutritional status of the subject at the time of collection; unfortunately, it does not always do so. In protein calorie malnutrition the tissues may be maintaining normal, or near normal, protein levels in the blood. This may happen despite inadequacy of the protein intake and even in the presence of clinical signs. Hemoconcentration in hot climates may result in blood nutrient values that are elevated and misleading. Sometimes the time of collection of the specimen affects the result.[101] The validity of the data also depends on the method used, the mode of collection of the specimen, and the standards of quality control in the laboratory. The values may be affected if the specimen is subjected to excessive shaking, heat, exposure to air or ultraviolet light, or the addition of preservatives.

Full details of tests that are used to evaluate nutritional adequacy can be found in standard laboratory texts and field manuals. Some specific tests used to evaluated certain deficiency states will be discussed in further detail.

Protein calorie malnutrition   So far, no laboratory has been able to produce a completely satisfactory biochemical test for malnutrition that is suitable for use in all parts of the world.[102] Many analytical procedures have been tested but their value is still unproven.

Calorie adequacy   An evaluation of calorie adequacy would require estimates of the Basal Metabolic Rate and estimates of energy expenditure (see page 243). This cannot be done on a sufficiently wide scale in routine nutritional surveys. Similarly, blood glucose, free fatty acid, and ketone body estimations, are not suitable for population studies. This means that the evaluation of calorie adequacy depends on anthropometrical measurements and dietary appraisal.

Protein adequacy Several tests are used and they are the subject of much controversy. Serum total protein and albumin levels do not fall below the normal range until late in the disease when clinical signs of malnutrition are starting to appear. The changes, even then, may be restricted to the kwashiorkor type of case since many cases of marasmus have levels within normal ranges. Hookworm infestation affects protein metabolism in protein deficient children, consequently, the total serum levels may be extremely low. Infections stimulate an increase in serum globulins which inflate total serum protein levels. The effects of infestation and infection can not always be assessed in nutrition surveys; even mean values of serum protein levels in communities may not be suitable for comparative purposes.

Urinary urea-creatinine ratio Low ratios are found in subjects consuming low protein diets, thus the ratio is a measure of the intake of protein rather than nutritional status. It should, be used therefore, in conjunction with dietary studies where it may serve as a cross-check. If the glomerular filtration rate is increased, the excretion of urea is increased but creatinine excretion is not affected. On first rising, the glomerular filtration rate usually increases. To avoid spurious tests, the first urine voided in the morning should be discarded.

Urinary sulfur-creatinine ratio This is a similar test to the urea-creatinine test but it has the advantage of reflecting the intake of protein containing sulfur amino acids, usually associated with proteins of high biological value.

Serum amino acid ratio The essential and non-essential amino acid levels in serum can be estimated without undue technical difficulty. It has been noted that the ratio of non-essential to essential amino acids is disturbed in protein calorie malnutrition. The serum amino acid ratio is determined from the non-essential amino acids, glycine, serine, glutamine, and taurine, and the essential amino acids, leucine, isoleucine, valine, and methionine. Normally, the ratio of non-essential to essential amino acids is less than 2. Values of over 4 are found in kwashiorkor. While high ratios may be a true reflection of protein deficiency, lower values do not mean that malnutrition does not exist and the test should always be considered in relation to other criteria. Unfortunately, the test has proved to be of value only where the main nutritional deficiency is protein. In those areas where there is general undernutrition, the test is too unreliable to have practical value. Even in protein deficiency, it tends to be unreliable because the recent intake of protein can influence the amino acid patterns. Fasting samples of serum may obviate this difficulty.

Urinary hydroxyproline index Hydroxyproline is a product of collagen metabolism. In protein calorie malnutrition collagen metabolism is depressed. On this basis, it has been assumed that low levels of hydroxyproline excretion in the urine may be a feature of protein deficiency. When the total excretion is measured over 24 hours, the test is reliable. However, in community surveys it is impractical to collect urine samples over a whole day so the excretion has been related to the excretion of creatinine present in the same sample. It has been assumed that the two components are excreted in the same relative concentrations throughout the day, and that the level of hydroxyproline excretion does not materially alter with age. Minor daily flucations in excretion do occur but these are not sufficient to invalidate the result, but the excretion of hydroxyproline in childhood is not constant and it is affected by parasites and infections. The test should only be used to evaluate communities of children and more research is required before the hydroxyproline index can be considered a valid measure of malnutrition.

Urinary creatinine-height index In malnutrition, there is cessation of growth. There is also muscle wasting associated with a decrease in the excretion of creatinine. The decreased excretion of creatinine in relation to height may therefore be considered as an index of protein calorie malnutrition. The test is accurate over 24 hours but is impractical in the field. As glomerular filtration rates are not constant during the course of the day, the sample collected may not be truly representative of the 24 hour excretion of creatinine. Because of these problems, the test may have more value in evaluating recovery of malnourished children.

Although biochemical tests have limited use in the evaluation of protein calorie malnutrition, they should not be abandoned. Further research may produce more reliable methodologies. In the meantime, the value of the test is enhanced if other tests of nutrient levels are conducted at the same time. In all cases they should be correlated with clinical, dietary, and anthropometric observations.

Vitamin A This nutrient is stored in the liver and the reserves may be determined directly by liver biopsy. This procecure is not without danger and it should not be employed in community surveys. Because the protein deficient body is unable to mobilize stores of vitamin A, high storage levels should be interpreted with caution in areas where protein calorie malnutrition exists. Serum retinol levels reflect the dietary intake of vitamin A but not necessarily vitamin A activity since some of the forms of retinol are not utilized by the body.

Thiamine The excretion of thiamine in the urine seems to be linearly related to intake except at very low levels. Excretion is lowered in pregnancy In children the range of normality is less clear. Because of this, and the individual variation in thiamine excretion, it is recommended that the activity of the enzyme transketolase in red blood cells should also be measured.[103] This enzyme depends on thiamine so its activity is a direct measure of thiamine status. There are however, difficulties in interpreting erythrocyte transketolase (ETK) activity because great variations are found in normal subjects. It has recently been suggested that the measurement of the effects of giving thiamine pyrophosphate on the erythrocyte transketolase activity may be a better index of thiamine status. Research indicates that if the ETK activity is greatly increased, the result is indicative of beri-beri. The practical difficulties in conducting the test precludes its use in community surveys.[104] The effect of loading the body with the vitamin and measuring the excretion may give an index of deficiency but again the test is impracticable in community surveys. The measurement of accumulation of pyruvic acid (a metabolite that appears in thiamine deficiency) is also too elaborate for field surveys.

Niacin Levels of niacin in tissues do not always reflect the clinical course of pellagra. Metabolites of niacin are excreted in the urine and are measurable. In field surveys the simple estimation of N'-methylnicotinamide per gram of creatinine in random urine specimens gives useful information which may corroborate dietary data.

Riboflavin The levels of riboflavin in blood can be measured accurately but it has been concluded that the amount of free riboflavin in blood is too variable to serve as a useful index of riboflavin nutriture. As riboflavin excretion in the urine is related to the intake, estimates of urinary riboflavin in a single fasting specimen of urine may be used to assess the status of adult levels. In children, the test may be unreliable as their needs and consumption are greater and there are no established standards of reference for riboflavin excretion in children. A riboflavin load test, in which the excretion of urinary riboflavin is measured after ingesting 1 mg of the vitamin, is not yet practicable in field surveys.

Vitamin C The concentration of plasma ascorbic acid is probably a good reflection of vitamin C levels in other tissues. The concentration decreases rapidly when the body is deprived of vitamin C, and disappears completely after about 6 weeks of total deprivation. There may not be signs of scurvy by this time, consequently low vitamin C levels are not diagnostic of scurvy. Ascorbic acid levels in white blood cells are a good measure of ascorbic acid status when tissue levels are low, but it is usually not possible to apply this test in community surveys. Load tests may indicate that a subject is saturated with ascorbic acid but they are not indicative of unsaturation. This test also is impractical for field surveys.

Vitamin D   Vitamin D status cannot be judged from the dietary intake because the vitamin can be synthesized in the body. As vitamin D deficiency develops, blood levels of the enzyme serum alkaline phosphatase increase proportionately to the extent of the deficiency. While serum alkaline phosphatase levels are of value in advanced deficiency, it has doubtful use in detecting early deprivation, especially in children. It has been noted that enzyme levels may be normal in protein deficient infants suffering from rickets.[105]

In osteomalacia there is an increase in serum alkaline phosphatase levels while there is a decrease in serum calcium. The validity of the test is in doubt however, as increases in serum alkaline phosphatase levels can occur in other pathological conditions.

Iron   The sequence of iron depletion is shown in Figure 118. It is apparent that an early diagnosis of anemia cannot be made from the morphology of the red cell. The earliest deficiencies can be detected by measuring the

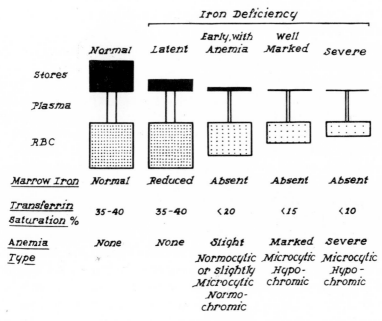

Figure 118   The sequence of iron depletion in man (Reproduced from *Clinical Hematology*, 6th Edition, by permission of Dr. M. M. Wintrobe and Lea and Febiger)

9*

iron in the stores, but this necessitates an examination of bone marrow, a painful procedure usually beyond the scope of a field survey team.

As iron deficiency develops, the plasma level of transferrin rises while the iron level falls (see page 292). This results in a decrease in the percentage of saturation of the transferrin. It is assumed that anemia is present if the saturation is less than 35 per cent. Unfortunately, a decrease in saturation also occurs in infections, chronic liver disease, and in protein calorie malnutrition. (It has been suggested that transferrin levels may be a good index of protein calorie nutritional status.[106]) However, at levels of less than 10 per cent saturation, the diagnosis of iron deficiency anemia is not in doubt.

The volume of packed red corpuscles can be determined by the *hematocrit*. It affords the same kind of information as the red cell count or hemoglobin estimation. In practice, most diagnoses of iron deficiency anemia are made by estimating hemoglobin levels in blood. Before discussing the accuracy, advantages, and disadvantages of different methods of estimating hemoglobin levels, it should be appreciated that possibly the greatest potential source of error lies in the collection of the blood sample. Venous blood is ideal for hemoglobin estimations but it may not be possible to collect venous blood under field conditions. Consequently the finger or heel is pricked and a small amount of blood (usually 0.02–0.05 ml) is withdrawn. The accurate measurement of such small amounts requires considerable skill. In addition, the concentration of the sample will be diluted if pressure is applied to the finger to assist the flow of blood because the process of squeezing adds lymph to the specimen. In many cases, accuracy depends on the quality of the pipettes. Hemoglobin pipettes sold on the open market may carry a calibration error of 5 per cent.

The methods used to measure hemoglobin levels are of three main types: those that involve chemical analysis of iron, those that measure the pigments in the blood, and those that measure the physical properties of blood.

These procedures involve the utilization of instruments and equipment that range from the very simplest of devices to highly complex and expensive electrophotometers. The accuracy of the results obtained varies between 50 per cent down to less than one-half of one per cent. The range of accuracy is not related however, to the cost of the equipment. For field work some inexpensive methods provide reliable and accurate data.

Instruments that measure hemoglobin levels are designated hemoglobinometers. The simplest is the *Tallqvist* which consists of a series of standard colors printed on a chart. Undiluted blood is collected on absorbent paper and the color of the "blot" is compared with these. The margin of error is between 20 and 50 per cent. Other hemoglobinometers compare colors, measure the optical density of diluted blood or measure the absorption of light as it passes through the blood.

The iron of the hemoglobin molecule can be detached and measured by comparison with the color of a standard solution of known iron content. In using this method, it is assumed that all of the iron in the blood is hemoglobin iron. This is not strictly correct as the plasma contains 0.4 per cent of the total iron in normal blood.

Hemoglobin may be converted into oxyhemoglobin, acid hematin, alkali hematin, cyanmethemoglobin, cyanhematin. The pigment is then measured visually or by photoelectric methods.

The oldest methods of measuring oxyhemoglobin used diluted blood that was then matched with a standard chemical solution or a colored glass standard. One of the modern hemoglobinometers uses transmitted green light to compare the sample with a variable standard. The conversion of hemoglobin to acid hematin is the basis of the *Sahli* test. The addition of water to the blood sample is not only tedious, but, if too much is added, the test has to be repeated. Acid hematin also becomes darker on standing. This is not a serious drawback if the test is carried out after ten minutes when most of the pigment has formed. Standards are not always reliable and the test is subject to "observer" errors. An additional inaccuracy arises because some of the hemoglobin may not be converted to acid hematin. This difficulty is overcome by converting the hemoglobin to alkali hematin. In the newborn, this method has its drawbacks because fetal hemoglobin (present in the young infant) is not converted to alkali hematin.

Ferricyanide can be used to convert the hemoglobin to cyanmethemoglobin. The optical density of the blood diluted by the ferricyanide solution is measured optically. Cyanhematin can also be prepared and its color intensity may be measured either visually or photoelectrically. This method has a high degree of accuracy.

The physical properties of blood can also be measured in several ways. The oxygen capacity of the blood may be determined. The method is accurate but it is time consuming and requires expensive apparatus. The specific gravity may be measured very easily by dropping blood into serial dilutions of copper sulphate. The drop will remain suspended when the specific gravity of the copper sulphate is the same as the blood. A nomogram can be used to convert the specific gravity of the blood to grams of hemoglobin.[107] The test may be simplified for screening populations by using one strength of copper sulphate representing a level below which anemia is said to be present. A drop of whole blood floating or suspended in this solution would signify anemia, a drop that sinks would signify normality.

Vitamin B_{12}   Deficiency of vitamin B_{12} is usually confirmed by development of megaloblastic anemia. Occult vitamin B_{12} deficiency is believed to be much more common than previously supposed suggesting the need for a community screening test. So far only two procedures are in use. The first detects serum antibodies to the gastric parietal cells that secrete the intrinsic factor. The second involves a microbiological estimation of the vitamin in serum. These techniques call for specialized equipment, a supply of normal stomach tissue, and special skills. This renders them impracticable for use in nutrition surveys.[108]

Iodine   The excretion of iodine in urine samples collected in goitrous regions is much lower than the excretion of iodine in non-goitrous areas. This test cannot be applied on an individual basis because the excretion of iodine is subject to many influences. The amount of iodine bound to serum proteins is a useful measure of the functional state of the thyroid gland but for surveys it is not valid because in endemic goiter patients frequently have normal thyroid function. Low levels are also found in apparently normal children.

Biochemical assessment of the status of iodine nutrition may have no advantage over the physical appraisal of the thyroid gland.

The relevance of biochemical assessment of nutritional status is unquestioned but it is obvious that many of the tests are impracticable for field work. A comment made some years ago by Albanese and Orto[109] is still pertinent. "In the light of the concept of nutritional individuality, it is doubtful if the precision attained by elaborate techniques is meaningful, or useful, in resolving problems of practical nutrition."

Biophysical assessment of nutritional status

Very little use is made of the physical properties of tissues and much research is needed on this potentially important aspect of nutritional assessment. Tissues such as the skin, hair, nails, buccal mucous membrane, and teeth are readily accessible. There are a variety of physical tests that can be applied to some, or all of them, including hardness, strength, extensibility, brittleness, electrical conductivity, reaction to chemical dyes and stains. Other tissues such as bone, may be examined radiologically. The tissues of the central nervous system may be tested for reflex activity, the muscles for performance. The circulatory system may be tested for changes in hydrostatic and hydrodynamic characteristics and the blood vessels for fragility. In Chapter 1, attention was drawn to neurological disorders including nerve deafness which featured a clinical syndrome of vitamin B inadequacy. This indicates a need for tests of fingertip sensation and perhaps hearing tests in areas where this syndrome may be prevalent.[110] One of the other senses, vision, is frequently tested in areas where vitamin A deficiency is prevalent.

Dark Adaption   Vitamin A deficiency leads to night blindness (*hemeralopia*). Normally, when a healthy person enters a dark room from the light, there is a period of temporary blindness but in the space of a few minutes the sight adapts to the reduced light intensity. In night blindness this adaptation takes much longer because there is inadequate vitamin A for the formation of rhodopsin. Several "adaptometers" for measuring dark adaptation have been used but studies have revealed that dark adaptation may be impaired for non-nutritional reasons. The use of the test in surveys is, therefore, of limited value. In addition to this serious drawback, the test is not easy to carry out on young children who may be the group most "at risk".

Nail   Nail has a growth rate influenced by nutritional status but estimation of growth is laborious and impractical. It has been argued that, as the structure of the nail is affected by malnutrition, its physical properties might be affected similarly. Nails from malnourished populations have been found to be harder than nails from healthy, well nourished populations.[111] Much more research is required to verify these preliminary reports but if hardness does increase in malnutrition the test could have value in screening communities.

Hair   In protein calorie malnutrition this material shows gross changes in pigmentation, brittleness, tensile strength and pluckability. Significant differences have been reported in the tensile strength of hair in malnourished children compared with well nourished children of the same race.[112] While the specimens are relatively easy to collect, the measurement of tensile strength is a procedure that would be beyond the scope of most laboratories in developing countries.

A reduction in hair diameter has also been reported in malnutrition and serial measurements of the hair are believed to reflect the nutritional history of the patient. It has also been noticed that the period of time over which narrowing takes place is longer than the duration of illness.[113] This suggests that the test could be used to detect pre-clinical kwashiorkor. Changes in the morphology of hair root have also been reported in malnutrition.[114]

The hair shafts become brittle, they lack pigment, the roots show atrophy and the internal and external hair root sheaths are absent. The percentage of hairs in the growth stage is less than that found in normal children.

During protein repletion, the hair reverts back to normal. Although imperfect sheaths are formed at first, later they become complete and the hair bulb returns to its normal size and form.

The test may have considerable value in the rapid evaluation of the nutritional status of a population but further research will be required to determine whether significant changes can be detected in mild cases of protein calorie malnutrition.

Buccal mucous membrane   The buccal mucous membrane is a tissue that can be used as biopsy material. Scrapings of the mucosa from inside the mouth can be stained to show the cytoplasmic characteristics of the cells.[115] The reaction of the cells to the stain depends on the time that they take to mature. Shortening of the maturation period occurs in protein calorie deficiency, infection, and old age, and can be detected on microscopic examination of stained smears. It has been suggested that the test may be employed as a simple screening procedure. However, a recent field evaluation of the procedure has cast doubts on its validity as mildly malnourished children showed fewer cytological changes than the well nourished group.[116]

Electrocardiography   The cardiac output is reduced in severe protein calorie malnutrition. This has been attributed to myocardial damage and potassium and magnesium deficiency. The disturbed function can be detected by the electrocardiograph.[117,118]

Transillumination of the skull   The effects of malnutrition on brain growth are most marked during the first few months of life when proliferation of the cells of the nervous system is at a peak. It is known that the head diameter of marasmic infants is less than that of the well fed. In severe cases there may be a definite brain atrophy with a consequent disproportion between the size of the brain and the skull. The space between the brain and the skull is filled with fluid that can be detected by transilluminating the head with a powerful light. Normally the area of transillumination around the light source is approximately 2 cm wide. In severe cases of marasmus the area of transillumination may extend over the whole of the dome of the skull.[119] This technique has not been assessed in the field (see plate 23).

Radiography   Radiography may be used to measure soft tissue thickness, the character of the bone, the function of the heart and circulatory system, and the gastrointestinal tract.

The role of radiography in measuring soft tissue thickness and delays in ossification has already been described.

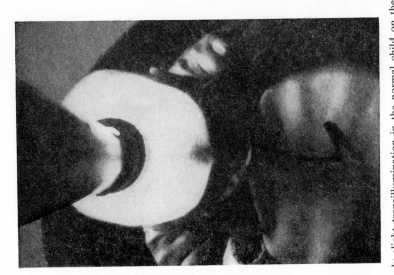

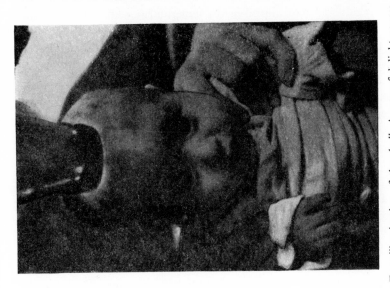

Plate 23   Transillumination of the skull. A powerful light causes only slight transillumination in the normal child on the left. When fluid is present between the brain and the skull in malnutrition there is a large area of transillumination (right). (Photographs supplied by Dr. Fernando Monckeberg B)

Radiographs of the long bones may reveal changes characteristic of lead poisoning. Lines of arrest which have been attributed to nutritional causes may be seen in malnutrition but they may also occur in infections and growth arrest caused by hormonal imbalance.[120]

In protein calorie malnutrition, radiography may reveal a loss of compact bone in the limbs and reduction in the thickness of the skull bones.[121]

Changes in the radiological appearance of bone are also observed in osteomalacia. These typically include *pseudo-fractures* but the detection of small degrees of decalcification may not be possible. The enlargement of the wrists and osteochondral junctions in rickets are also apparent on radiographs.

In fluorosis there is increased density of bones and thickening of its cortex. Calcification of ligaments may be observed and bony outgrowths may be seen on the spine.[122]

In infantile scurvy there is a loss of density of long bones and *lines of arrest* may be seen on the tibia.

Enlargement of the heart is a feature of cardiac beri-beri in adults, but it is probably rare in the infantile form of the disease. In protein calorie malnutrition, cardiomegaly is reported but as the heart size before the onset of malnutrition is usually unknown, the enlargement cannot be attributed conclusively to malnutrition. In undernutrition there is a reduction of heart size but the diagnosis of undernutrition cannot be based on radiography unless a previous x-ray is available for comparison.

In kwashiorkor the lung field may be hypertranslucent or hypertransradiant and there may be pulmonary hypovascularity.[123]

Distended loops of bowel and multiple fluid levels are a common feature of protein calorie malnutrition and they appear early in the disease.[124] While radiography may confirm the presence of disease, its main use in field surveys is restricted at present, to the evaluation of delay in ossification.

Animal feeding experiments Laboratory animals may be used to evaluate diets consumed by human populations. Rats are omnivorous and may be fed diets incorporating components identical in proportion to those in the human diet. The experiment should include a control group of rats fed adequate protein and calories equivalent to the calorie level of the experimental groups. Table 80 shows an evaluation of two Indonesian diets.

The preceeding pages have outlined the *epidemiological approach* to the assessment of the nutritional status of individuals and communities. An examination of past experience shows however, that surveys, or inquiries

Table 80 The protein value of two Javanese diets

Type of diet	Calories per 100 g	Average food intake (g)	Average growth-increment (%)	Average NPU_{op}	Average N_2 Cont. of Diet (%)	Protein Nx 5.95 (%)	Protein Cal. %	NDpCal%
I (West Java)	380	308.2	22.2	56	1.18	7.02	7.4	4.2
II (East Java)	386	301.4	28.4	59	1.49	8.86	9.6	5.4
Control	410	247.7	30.4	75	1.57	10.00*	10.0	7.4

* Nx 6.38

Source: Van Veen, A. G., Hong, L. G., Nioe, O. K. *Ecol. Food and Nutr.* **1**: 39, 1971

into nutritional status usually have failed to stimulate remedial action. The inquiry should mark the beginning and not the end of nutrition activities. The next chapter will discuss how programs may be organized, and services delivered to prevent, control, and relieve malnutrition.

References

1. Jelliffe, D. B. *The Assessment of the Nutritional Status of the Community.* Monograph No. 53. World Health Organization, Geneva, 1966.
2. Bigwood, E. J. *Guiding Principles for Studies on the Nutrition of Populations.* League of Nations Geneva, 1939.
3. *Manual for Nutrition Surveys.* Second Edition. ICNND, National Institutes of Health, Bethesda, 1963.
4. Ferro, Luzzi G. "Rapid Evaluation of Nutritional Level." *Amer. J. Clin. Nutr.* **19**: 247, 1966.
5. Garrow, J. S., Smith, R., Ward, E. E. *Electrolyte Metabolism in Severe Infantile Malnutrition*, p. 4. London: Pergamon Press, 1968.
6. *Manual on Food and Nutrition Policy.* F. A. O. Nutritional Studies, No. 22, p. 15, F. A. O. Rome 1969.
7. *The State of Food and Agriculture 1968*, p. 11. F. A. O. Rome 1968.
8. *The State of Food and Agriculture 1957*, p. 77. F. A. O. Rome 1957.
9. *Manual on Food and Nutrition Policy.* F. A. O. Nutritional Studies, No. 22, p. 8, F. A. O. Rome 1969.
10. Rice, Grain of Life. World Food Problems. No. 6, F. A. O. Rome 1966.
11. Jelliffe, D. B. *The Assessment of the Nutritional Status of the Community.* Monograph No. 53, p. 60. World Health Organization, Geneva, 1966.

12. Wills, V. G., Waterlow, J. C. "The Death Rate in the Age Group 1-4 Years as an Index of Malnutrition." *J. Trop. Ped.* **4**: 167, 1958.

13. Gordon, J. E., Wyon, J. B., Ascoli, W. "The Second Year Death Rate in Less Developed Countries." *Amer. J. Med. Sci.* **254**: 357, 1967.

14. *International Classification of Diseases*, Vols. 1 and 2. World Health Organization, Geneva 1967 and 1969.

15. Behar, M., Ascoli, W., Scrimshaw, N. S. "An investigation Into the Cause of Death in Children in Four Rural Communities in Guatemala." Bull. W. H. O. **19**: 1093, 1958.

16. Reh, E. *Manual on Household Food Consumption Surveys.* F. A. O. Nutritional Studies, No. 18, F. A. O. Rome 1962.

17. Becker, B. G., Indik, B. P., Beeuwkes, A. M. *Dietary Intake Methodologies-A review.* University of Michigan, 1960.

18. Madhavan, S., Swaminathan, M. C. A Comparative Study of Two Methods of Diet Survey." *Indian J. Med. Res.* **54**: 480, 1966.

19. Abramson, J. H., Slome, G., Kosovsky, G. "Food Frequency Interview as an Epidemiological Tool." *Amer. J. Public Health* **53**: 1093, 1963.

20. Chassy, J. P., van Veen, A. G., Young, F. W. "The Application of Social Science Research Methods to the Study of Food Habits and Food Consumption in an Industrializing Area." *Amer. J. Clin. Nutr.* **20**: 56, 1967.

21. Watt, B. K., Merrill, A. L. *Composition of Foods.* Agricultural Handbook No. 8, United States Department of Agriculture, Washington, D. C. 1963.

22. Platt, B. S. Tables of Representative Values of Foods Commonly Used in Tropical Countries. Medical Research Council, Special Report Series No. 302, H. M. S. O., London 1965.

23. McCance, R. A., Widdowson, E. M. The Composition of Foods. Medical Research Council, Special Report Series No. 297, H. M. S. O., London 1969.

24. *Amino Acid Content of Food.* F. A. O. Nutritional Studies No. 24, F. A. O. Rome, 1970.

25. McCance, R. A., Widdowson, E. M. The Composition of Foods. Medical Research Council, Special Report Series No. 297, H. M. S. O., London 1969.

26. Walker, A. R. P. "Nutritional, Biochemical and Other Studies on South African Populations." *S. Afr. Med. J.* **40**: 814, 1966.

27. McCance, R. A., Widdowson, E. M. The Composition of Foods. Medical Research Council, Special Report Series No. 297, p. 162, H. M. S. O., London 1969.

28. Deyoe, C. W., Shellenburger, J. A. "Amino Acids or Proteins in Sorghum Grain." *J. Agri. Food Chem.* **13**: 446, 1965.

29. Somogyi, J. C., Schiele, K. "Der Vitamin-C-Gehalt verschiedener Kartoffelsorten und seine Abnahme während der Lagerung." *Int. J. Vit. Res.* **36**: 337, 1966.

30. Eagles, J. A., Whiting, M. G., Olson, R. E. "Dietary Appraisal. Problems in Processing Dietary Data." *Amer. J. Clin. Nutr.* **19**: 1, 1966.

31. Widdowson, E. M. "How the Foetus is Fed." *Proc. Nutr. Soc.* **28**: 17, 1969.

32. Antonov, A. N. "Children Born During the Siege of Leningrad in 1942." *J. Pediat.* **30**: 250, 1947.

33. Smith, C. A. "The Effect of War-time Starvation in Holland Upon Pregnancy and Its Products." *Amer. J. Obstet. and Gynecol.* **53**: 599, 1947.

34. Osofsky, H. J. "Antenatal Malnutrition. Its Relationship to Subsequent Infant and Child Development." *Amer. J. Obstet and Gynecol.* **105**: 1150, 1969.

35. Platt. B. S., Stewart, R. J. C. "Effect of Protein-Calorie Deficiency in Dogs." *Develop. Med. and Child Neurol.* **10:** 3, 1968.
36. Blackwell, B. N., Blackwell, R. Q., Yu, T. T. S., Weng, Y. C., Chow, B. F. "Further Studies on Growth and Feed Utilization in Progeny of Underfed Mother Rats." *J. Nutr.* **97:** 79, 1969.
37. Winick, M., Rosso, P. "Head Circumference and Cellular Growth of the Brain in Normal and Marasmic Infants." *J. Pediat.* **74:** 774, 1969.
38. Burke, B. S., Harding, V. V., Stuart, H. C. "Nutrition Studies During Pregnancy." *J. Pediat.* **23:** 506, 1943.
39. Jeans, P. C., Smith, M. B., Stearns, G. J. "Incidence of Prematurity in Relation to Maternal Nutrition." *J. Amer. Diet. Assoc.* **31:** 576, 1955.
40. Latham, M. C., Robson, J. R. K. "Birthweight and Prematurity." *Trans. Roy. Soc. Trop. Med. Hyg.* **60:** 791, 1966.
41. Valtuena, Borgue O. "Weight of Newborn Infants in Madrid as an Index of Nutritional State of the Population." *Rev. Espanola Pediat.* **22:** 147, 1966.
42. Usher, R., McLean, F. "Intrauterine Growth of Live-born Caucasian Infants at Sea Level." *J. Pediat.* **74:** 901, 1969.
43. Donald, I. "Sonar as a Method of Studying Prenatal Development." *J. Pediat.* **75:** 326, 1969.
44. Hellman, L. M., Kobayashi, M., Fillisti, L., Lavenlaf, M., Cromb, E. "Growth and Development of the Human Fetus Prior to the Twentieth Week of Gestation." *Amer. J. Obstet. and Gynecol.* **103:** 789, 1969.
45. Robson, J. R. K. "Seasonal Influences on Height and Weight Increments of Boys and Girls in Tanganyika." *J. Trop. Med. Hyg.* **67:** 46, 1964.
46. Dawkins, M. J., Hull, D. "The Production of Heat by Fat." *Sci. Amer.* **213:** 62, August 1965.
47. Hirsch, J., Knittle, J. L. "Cellularity of Obese and Non-Obese Human Adipose Tissue." *Fed. Proc.* **29:** 1516, 1970.
48. Cheek, D. B., Hill, D. E. "Muscle and Liver Cell Growth: Role of Hormones and Nutritional Factors." *Fed. Proc.* **29:** 1503, 1970.
49. Garn, S. M., Rohman, C. G. Interaction of Nutrition and Genetics in the Timing of Growth and Development, p. 353, Vol. 13, *Pediatric Clinics of North America.* Philadelphia: W. B. Saunders, 1966.
50. Craig, J. W. "Present Knowledge of Nutrition in Inborn Errors of Metabolism." *Nutr. Rev.* **26:** 161, 1968.
51. Thomson, A. M. "Maternal Stature and Reproductive Efficiency." *Eugen Rev.* **51:** 157, 1959.
52. Tanner, J. M. *Education and Physical Growth*, p. 116. University of London Press, 1961.
53. Ito, P. K. "Comparative Biometrical Study of Physique of Japanese Women Born and Reared Under Different Environments." *Human Biol.* **14:** 279, 1942.
54. Walker, A. R. P., de Lacey, C. D. "Growth, Nutrition and Parasitism." *Trans. Roy. Soc. Trop. Med. Hyg.* **56:** 173, 1962.
55. Smith, D. W. "Compendium of Shortness of Stature." *J. Pediat.* **70:** 465, 1967.
56. Gesell, A., Amatruda, C. S. Environmental Retardation, p. 316. In *Developmental Diagnosis*, 2nd Ed. New York: Hoeber, 1951.
57. Spitz, R. A. "Hospitalism." The Psychoanalytic Study of the Child. **1:** 53, 1945.
58. Lowrey, L. G. "Personality Distortion and Early Institutional Care." *Amer. J. Orthopsych.* **10:** 576, 1940.

59. Bakwin, H. "Emotional Deprivation in Infants." *J. Pediat.* **35:** 512, 1949.
60. Talbot, N. B., Sobel, E. H., Burke, B. S., Lineman, E., Kautman, S. B. "Dwarfism in Healthy Children, Its Possible Relation to Emotional, Nutritional and Endocrine Disturbances." *New Eng. J. Med.* **236:** 783, 1947.
61. Widdowson, E. M. "Mental Contentment and Physical Growth." *The Lancet* **1:** 1316, 1951.
62. Coleman, R., Provence, S. A. "Developmental Retardation in Infants Living in Families." *Pediatrics* **19:** 285, 1957.
63. Barbero, G. J., Shaheen, E. "Environmental Failure to Thrive, A Clinical View." *J. Pediat.* **71:** 639, 1967.
64. Spaulding, J. S. "Growth and Development, the Challenge of Short Stature." *J. Kansas Med. Soc.* **69:** 118, 1968.
65. Glaser, K., Eisenberg, L. "Maternal Deprivation." *Pediatrics* **18:** 626, 1956.
66. Bullard, D. M., Glaser, H. H., Heagarty, M. C., Pivchik, E. C. "Failure to Thrive in the 'Neglected' Child." *Amer. J. Orthopsych.* **37:** 680, 1967.
67. Abramowicz, M. "Height of 12 Year Old Puerto Rican Boys in New York City: Origins in Difference." *Pediatrics* **43:** 427, 1969.
68. Michelson, N. "Studies in the Physical Development of Negroes; Onset of Puberty." *Amer. J. Phys. Anthropol.* **2:** 151, 1944.
69. Kark, E. "Menarche in South African Bantu Girls." *S. Afr. J. Med. Sci.* **8:** 35, 1943.
70. Kralj-Cercek, L. "The Influence of Food, Body Build, and Social Origin on Age at Menarche." *Human Biol.* **28:** 393, 1956.
71. Ellis, R. W. B. "Growth and Health of Belgian Children." *Arch. Dis. Childh.* **20:** 97, 1945.
72. Scott, J. A. Report on Heights and Weights of School Pupils in the County of London, 1959. London County Council 1961.
73. Wilson, D. C., Sutherland, I. "Age at the Menarche." *Brit. Med. J.* p. 1267, May 27, 1950.
74. Jelliffe, D. B. The Assessment of the Nutritional Status of the Community, Monograph No. 53, World Health Organization, Geneva, 1966.
75. *Manual for Nutrition Surveys.* Second Edition. ICNND National Institutes of Health, Bethesda, 1963.
76. Robson, J. R. K., Mather, F., Jones, E. L. "The Accuracy of Measurement of Weight in the Well-Baby Clinic." *J. Trop. Pediat.* **16:** 5, 1970.
77. Jelliffe, D. B. The Assessment of the Nutritional Status of the Community. Monograph No. 53, World Health Organization, Geneva, 1966.
78. Durnin, J. V. G. A., Rahaman, M. M. "The Assessment of the Amount of Fat in the Human Body from Measurements of Skinfold Thickness." *Brit. J. Nutr.* **21:** 681, 1967.
79. Young, C. M. "Predicting Body Fatness of Young Women on the Basis of Skinfold." *New York State J. of Med.* **62:** 1671, 1962.
80. Selzer, C. C., Mayer, J. "Simple Criterion of Obesity." *Postgrad. Med.* **38:** A101, 1965.
81. Robson, J. R. K., Bazin, M., Soderstrom, R. "Ethnic Differences in Skinfold Thickness." *Amer. J. Clin Nutr* **24:** 864, 1971.
82. Malina, R. M. "Patterns of Development in Skinfolds of Negro and White Philadelphia Children." *Human Biol.* **38:** 89, 1966.
83. Winick, M., Rosso, P. "Head Circumference and Cellular Growth of the Brain in Normal and Marasmic Infants." *J. Pediat.* **74:** 774, 1969.

84. Bray, P. F., Shields, W. D., Wolcott, G. J., Madsen, J. A. "Occipitofrontal Head Circumference, An Accurate Measure of Intracranial Volume." *J. Pediat.* **75**: 303 1969.
85. "The Arm Circumference as a Public Health Index of Protein-Calorie Malnutrition in Early Childhood," *J. Trop. Pediat.* **15**: 177, 1969.
86. Lagundoye, S. B., Reddy, S. "Chest X-Ray Changes in Kwashiorkor." *J. Trop. Pediat.* **16**: 124, 1970.
87. Garn, S. M., Rohman, C. G. "Variability in the Order of Ossification of the Bony Centers of the Hand and Wrist." *Amer. J. Phys. Anthropol.* **18**: 219, 1960.
88. Frisancho, A. R., Garn, S. M., Rohman, C. G. "Age at Menarche, A New Method of Prediction and Retrospective Assessment Based on Hand X-Rays." *Human Biol.* **41**: 42, 1969.
89. Morley, D. C. "Prevention of Protein Calorie Deficiency Syndromes." *Trans. Roy Soc. Trop. Med. Hyg.* **62**: 200, 1968.
90. Cuthbertson, W. J. F., Morley, D. C. "A Health and Weight Chart for Children from Birth to Five." *W. Afr. Med. J.* **11**: 237, 1962.
91. Gurney, J. M. "Anthropometry in Action (III) A Simple Tool for Assessing the Growth of School-Age Children." *J. Trop. Pediat.* **15**: 9, 1969.
92. Tanner, J. M., Whitehouse, R. H., Takaishi, M. "Standards from Birth to Maturity for Height, Weight, Height Velocity and Weight Velocity: British Children 1965," Part. II. *Arch. Dis. Childh.* **41**: 613, 1966.
93. Grant, M. W. *Technique for the Analysis of Height and Weight Data in Tropical Countries.* London School of Hygiene and Tropical Medicine, 1951.
94. *The Health Aspects of Food and Nutrition*, p. 285, World Health Organization, Manila, 1969.
95. Ford, F. J. "Can A Standard for 'Malnutrition' in Childhood be Devised?" *J. Trop. Pediat.* **10**: 47, 1964.
96. Jelliffe, D. B. The Assessment of the Nutritional Status of the Community. Monograph No. 53, World Health Organization, Geneva 1966.
97. *Manual for Nutrition Surveys.* Second Edition. ICNND National Institutes of Health, Bethesda, 1963.
98. Expert Committee on Medical Assessment of Nutritional Status. World Health Organization Technical Report Series No. 258, Geneva 1963.
99. Heard, C. R. C., Kriegsman, S. M., Platt, B. S. "The Interpretation of Plasma Amino Acid Ratios in Protein-Calorie Deficiency." *Brit. J. Nutr.* **23**: 203, 1969.
100. Truswell, A. S., Wanneburg, P., Wittman, W., Hansen, J. D. L. "Plasma-Amino Acids in Kwashiorkor." *The Lancet* **1**: 1162, 1966.
101. Young, V. R., Hussein, M. A., Murray, E., Scrimshaw, N. S. "Tryptophan Intake, Spacing of Meals, and Diurnal Fluctuations of Plasma Tryptophan in Men." *Amer. J. Clin. Nutr.* **22**: 1563, 1969.
102. Committee Report. "Assessment of Protein Nutritional Status." *Amer. J. Clin. Nutr.* **23**: 807, 1970.
103. Sauberlich, H. E. "Biochemical Alterations in Thiamine Deficiency—Their interpretation." *Amer. J. Clin. Nutr.* **20**: 528, 1967.
104. Tanphaichitr, V., Vimokesant, S. L., Dhanamitta, S., Valyasevi, A. "Clinical and Biochemical Studies of Adult Beri Beri." *Amer. J. Clin. Nutr.* **23**: 1017, 1970.
105. Reddy, V., Srikantia, S. G. "Serum Alkaline Phosphatase in Malnourished Children with Rickets." *J. Pediat.* **71**: 595, 1967.

106. McFarlane, H., Ogbeide, M. I., Reddy, S., Adcock, K. J., Adeshina, H., Gurney, J.M., Cooke, A., Taylor, G. O., Mordie, J. A. "Biochemical Assessment of Protein-Calorie Malnutrition." *The Lancet* **1**: 392, 1969.

107. Van Slyke, D. D., Philipps, R. A., Dole, V. P., Hamilton, B. P., Archibald, R. M., Plazin, J. "Calculations of Hemoglobin from Blood Specific Gravities." *J. Biol. Chem.* **183**: 349, 1950.

108. "Screening for Vitamin B_{12} Deficiency." *The Lancet* **2**: 310, 1969.

109. Albanese, A. A., Orto, L. A. Proteins and Amino Acids. In *Newer Methods of Nutritional Biochemistry*. New York: Academic Press, 1963.

110. Renfrew, S. "Fingertip Sensation." *The Lancet* **1**: 396, 1969.

111. Robson, J. R. K., el Tahawi, M. "The Hardness of Nail as an Index of Nutritional Status." *Brit. J. Nutr.* **26**: 233, 1971.

112. Latham, M. C., Velez, H. "The Tensile Strength of Hair in Protein-Calorie Malnutrition." *Proceedings, 7th International Congress on Nutrition, Hamburg.* **1**: 87, London: Pergamon Press, 1966.

113. Sims, R. T. "The Measurement of Hair Growth as an Index of Protein Synthesis in Malnutrition." *Brit. J. Nutr.* **22**: 229, 1968.

114. Bradfield, R. B., Bailey, M. A., Cordano, A. "Hair Root Changes in Andean Indian Children During Marasmic Kwashiorkor." *The Lancet* **2**: 1169, 1968.

115. Squires, B. T. "The Buccal Mucosa Cell Count in Health, Protein Calorie Deficiency, Infection and Old Age." *Cent. Afr. J. Med.* **12**: 223, 1966.

116. Wiersinga, A., Korte, R. "A Cytological Study on Buccal Smears as an Indicator of Nutritional Status." *E. Afr. Med. J.* **47**: 14, 1970.

117. Horsfall, P. A. L., Waldmann, E. "Electrocardiographic Changes in Kwashiorkor and Marasmus." *Cent. Afr. J. Med.* **14**: 170, 1968.

118. Khalil, M., El Khateeb, S., Kassem, S., Ellozy, M., Gabr, Y., Elwaseef, A. "Electrocardiographic Studies in Kwashiorkor." *J. Trop. Med. Hyg.* **72**: 291, 1969.

119. Fernando, Monckeberg B. The Effect of Malnutrition and Environment on Mental Development, p. 216. *Proceedings of Second Western Hemisphere Nutrition Congress 1968*. American Medical Association 1969.

120. Park, E. A. "The Imprinting of Nutritional Disturbance on the Growing Bone." *Pediatrics* **33**: Supple. 815, 1964.

121. Garn, S. M. Malnutrition and Skeletal Development in the Pre-school Child, p.43. In *Pre-school Child Malnutrition*. National Academy of Sciences Publication 1282, Washington, D. C. 1966.

122. Grech, P., Latham, M. C. "Fluorosis in the Northern Region of Tanganyika." *Trans. Roy. Soc. Trop. Med. Hyg.* **58**: 566, 1964.

123. Lagundoye, S. B., Reddy, S. "Chest X-Ray Changes in Kwashiorkor." *J. Trop. Ped.* **16**: 124, 1970.

124. Reichman, P., Stein, H. "Radiological Features Noted on Plain Radiographs in Malnutrition in African Children." *Brit. J. Radiol.* **41**: 296, 1968.

CHAPTER 6

Nutrition programs and services

In previous chapters, the nature and causation of global nutrition problems has been described and the reason for the disruption of normal body function by malnutrition has been discussed from a biological, chemical, and physiological standpoint. It should be apparent that the dysfunction is essentially a failure of an individual to meet his, or her, nutrient requirements. The reasons for this failure are numerous and interrelated. When a large number of people are affected, the resultant malnutrition presents a public health problem. The discussion which follows is concerned with the promotion of adequate nutrition, the prevention of malnutrition, and the management of overt malnutrition in the community. These basic objectives are achieved through the establishment of programs, "plans of procedure or systems under which action may be taken towards these desired goals", and services, "the action that furthers this purpose" (Webster's Dictionary).

The discussion is in four parts. The first deals with the planning, organization, and execution of nutrition programs. The second reviews existing programs and services. The third section will be devoted to an examination of nutrition services that meet special needs. The last section will discuss the problems of evaluation.

Planning nutrition programs

Although a nutrition program may be applied to individual communities, it is usual to consider nutritional problems on a wider basis and, for present purposes, attention will be focused on National Nutrition Programs and Services. The word "National" implies that the government has the prime responsibility and, so far as planning and administering a national nutrition program, this is true. When, however, the provision of services is concerned, it is obviously advantageous to utilize all possible resources so nutrition services may utilize private, or voluntary foundations and organizations.

The involvement of private voluntary services in a national plan introduces administrative complications. This is only one of many reasons why nutrition programs and services vary so much in emphasis, objectives, and organization.

It would very much simplify the task of planners of nutrition programs if there was a model nutrition program that could be adapted to conditions in various countries; unfortunately such a model does not exist. The reasons for this will be discussed in detail.

The planning, organization, and execution of a nutrition program depends on many factors including human behavior, technical considerations, administrative necessities, or established organizational procedures which are a legacy of health, or health-related programs.

In Chapter 1, *nutrition*, *malnutrition*, and *food* were defined; in practice these terms are interpreted differently by individual nations, governments, professional personnel, and the public. Even within one country, the interpretations vary from discipline to discipline, and between one government department and another. Frequently *nutrition* is synonymous with *food*, and *malnutrition* with *food inadequacy*. It is not surprising therefore to find a widespread assumption that malnutrition will be solved by the provision of food. Many nutrition programs are essentially food distribution programs that may be only putting a dressing on what is in reality a cancer.[1]

From time to time, new discoveries are made in the field of medicine and health which may have considerable social, political, and economic implications. For example, an inborn error of metabolism which causes the disease *phenylketonuria* in infants had a considerable impact on public health programs in the United States. The disease was first described in Germany in 1934.[2] After the discovery of a suitable test for the detection of cases some 28 years later,[3] programs were established in many parts of the United States for the identification of infants with persistently elevated blood phenylalanine concentrations.[4] Now, considerable sums of money and personnel are absorbed in detecting infants and children with phenylketonuria. Recently the justification for spending large sums of money on such programs has been questioned. In the State of Massachusetts for example, it has been pointed out that the examination of 277,644 children has revealed only 35 cases of phenylketonuria.[5]

Inappropriate planning of nutrition programs may be caused by inadequacy of data, and the failure to use existing data. In many countries there is a lack of basic information required to plan programs and services. Even in the United States, the nutritional status of the population is largely unknown.[6] In such circumstances it is not surprising that existing programs are the target of criticism.

Nutrition surveys have been carried out in many countries but in some of these the socio-economic and nutritional status of the population changed significantly while the results were being processed and published. The conclusions were valid for a previous period but their application may be inappropriate at a later time.

In recent years the trend towards laboratory research and detailed investigation of specific nutritional problems has provided vast amounts of data and information. Much of this cannot be used because it does not relate to conditions in the field. For example, detailed analyses of the nutrient content of raw foods have been made but there is very little information on the nutritive value of food *as prepared and consumed.* The planning of nutrition programs may depend on the calculation of nutrient intakes. If the raw food values alone are computed, the synergistic and antagonistic effects of nutrients in mixtures of foods may be missed. Any erroneous conclusions may be reflected in food and nutrition policies.

In earlier chapters it has been stressed that it is impossible to plan realistic and appropriate programs until the ecology of the situation is understood. In many countries however, existing data relating to ecology are ignored by scientific leaders who continue to give undue attention to "hard" data. While the need for objectivity is undisputed, it is impractical to wait until data of scientifically acceptable quality are available. It is unjustified also to formulate plans from data of unquestioned quality but not representative of the overall situation.

The basic problems that impede coordinated national planning have secondary effects. The limited understanding of the causation of malnutrition may have led to the development of food distribution programs. Food distribution programs utilizing surplus products have a dual purpose. The first is to support the market price of specified agricultural products and the second to supply food to malnourished individuals. The requirements of the two sectors of the country may not have a common basis. Agricultural products in need of price support may not be the products which supply the missing nutrients.

Programs designed to supply foods directly, or indirectly through the provision of money to purchase food, necessarily include rules and regulations which determine the eligibility of recipients to the program. The enforcement of inflexible eligibility regulations may deny the service to those who do not fit into prescribed categories but who may, nevertheless, be most in need of assistance.[7]

Laboratory research is frequently the product of universities and other institutes of learning. The data are more readily accepted by academicians

10*

because of its greater scientific value than field research which may lack experimental control. The academicians are responsible for moulding professionals and a new generation of professionals, highly trained in scientific reasoning, have taken over the leadership in program planning in many countries. However, their education and background may not have enabled them to achieve an understanding of the human problems existing in malnourished communities.

Technically advanced countries train, and educate, large numbers of professionals from developing countries. Unless care is taken, the student from overseas becomes oriented towards the problems of the affluent and is ill-prepared for the problems existing in his own country. Consequently, there is a real danger that on his return home there is a carry-over of influence from the sophisticated society that then affects program development in his own country.

The visitor to African and Asia will see numerous examples of expensive prestige projects in the field of nutrition mimicking those of the western world, but having little practical significance. Moreover, they divert funds, manpower, and time from more pressing, mundane problems. In addition to prestige projects, time and money may be spent also on activities that could be more appropriately and effectively executed in the western world.

While the theoretical planning of nutrition programs is far from easy, the execution of these plans is even more difficult. As an example, the needs of Pakistan will be examined.

Although villagers are the main food producers in Pakistan, they are often the worst fed. There are several reasons for this; first, the farmer may be growing an inadequate variety of food. He may be selling food but the proceeds may not be sufficient to allow him to purchase an adequate diet for his family. He may not, in fact, know what constitutes an adequate diet. There may be deficiencies in the food marketing and food distribution system so he may be unable to procure foods growing elsewhere in abundance. There is obviously a need for an agricultural program that will improve farming methods including crop yields, livestock breeding, and fish breeding. An efficient marketing and retail system is also required to allow food commodities to be purchased where they are needed.

In order to achieve these objectives, agronomists, cooperative and marketing specialists would be needed. The lack of knowledge regarding adequate diets calls for education through schools and agriculture extension. Teaching of nutrition in schools and colleges is frequently fragmented and contradictory which points out a need for unification of the content of the education offered in nutrition.

Population pressures are encroaching on available land indicating a need for population planning. Clinical surveys revealed widespread deficiencies in protein, vitamins, and minerals. Anemia, protein deficiency, goiter, keratomalacia, avitaminosos A, riboflavin deficiency, rickets, scurvy, and osteomalacia are common.[8] With this plethora of disease, it is obvious that the health and medical authorities must be concerned with the detection, prevention, control, and management of malnutrition as well as the usual programs for the control of communicable disease.

The number of disciplines involved in improving nutritional status is considerable even in this situation but in industrialized countries people live longer, so due attention has to be given to other health and nutritional problems associated with chronic disease conditions. There are also the problems of affluence, such as obesity and cardiovascular disease. The presence of these problems has led to the development of *categorical* programs and services, which may be absorbing sums of money and personnel quite out of proportion to the number of people affected. Each one of these categories may employ medical, health, and nursing personnel working independently of one another and with considerable autonomy within one department. Despite this, most health authorities have inadequacies in their services and it may be necessary to utilize existing resources more appropriately. It may be necessary to secure the collaboration of professionals, administrators, and subordinate staff within each of the disciplines and attempt to fit them into an overall program.

So far this has been viewed from the purely selfish view of nutrition. In reality, a country is faced with a series of health problems and it may be necessary to integrate nutrition into an overall health plan. The administrative complexities and magnitude of health problems in any community suggests that organization may be impossible. There is however, amidst all the confusion and misdirection of effort, clear indications of a path that might be followed. The theoretical rules and methods of procedure are relatively simple and a system for developing national nutrition programs and services will now be described. There are certain basic criteria; the first is central control and organization of the nutrition program. The second is an assured coordination of all the departments or ministries concerned with food or nutrition and the third is assured interdisciplinary collaboration and coordination, within the departments.

Central organization of nutrition programs and services

Study of the functions of the central organization helps to delineate the scope and character of the nutrition policy. In industrialized nations, the functions of the central organization are very numerous but underlying these there are some basic considerations. As the functions are identical and more clearly seen in developing countries, an uncomplicated ministerial system will be used as an example. Basic functions will be defined and the responsibility for fulfilling this function will be assigned to the appropriate administrative body (see Table 81)

Table 81   Functions and Ministerial responsibilities to nutrition

Function	Departmental or Ministerial responsibilities	
	Primary	Secondary
Agricultural production targets	Agriculture	Health, commerce, trade, co-operatives, marketing, community development
Food preservation and distribution	Agriculture	Health, marketing, trade, commerce, cooperatives, communications
Food Industrialization	Agriculture	Health, commerce, trade, community development, labor
Food enrichment	Health	Agriculture, industry, marketing, commerce
International trade	Agriculture	Trade, commerce, health
Social and Economic Policy	Health	community development, commerce, labor, education
Food consumption	Health	Agriculture, community development, cooperatives, commerce, trade, executive of central committee
Financing of programs and services	Finance	National Planning Board
Coordination	Executive of Central Committee	

Meeting agricultural production targets   This is, of course, the prime responsibility of the Ministry of Agriculture. In order to insure that food production targets are adequately orientated towards the nutritional needs of the country, the Ministry of Health must have responsibility for advising on what nutrients are needed. A joint decision has to be reached on which foods would help to meet the nutritional and agricultural needs of the country. The policy may affect the production of an export crop, or a cash crop, that may be an important source of revenue. The economic implications of changing existing food policies should be studied by the Ministries representing Commerce and Trade. If the policy is adopted and more produce becomes available, marketing problems may arise. These will have to be handled by the Ministries of Cooperative Development and Marketing. The produce may be new and unfamiliar to some communities and it may be necessary to seek the assistance of the Ministry of Community Development to facilitate its acceptability by the public.

Food processing, preservation and distribution   Surplus food may have to be stored, or converted into a state that will maintain its wholesomeness. At appropriate times, it will have to be distributed. It should be offered to the public free from any injurious preservatives, insecticides, or antibiotics. This function is the concern of the Ministry of Health. However, other Ministries responsible for the control of marketing and retail prices should also be involved. Finally, the whole success of a distribution system aiming to make surplus food commodities, or new agricultural products, available to the needy will depend on good communications. The Ministry of Public Works must therefore try to insure that the distribution system does not break down through failures in road or rail systems.

Food industrialization   Cereal foods produced in large quantities may stimulate the development of food industries. The problems caused by the consumption of highly refined cereal flours have already been described. It is undeniable however, that some food products, (cassava), may attract foreign trade and much needed foreign currency. The industries may employ a large work force. A compromise solution that pays due attention to the needs of business, as well as health, has to be reached between the Ministries of Health, Commerce and Trade, and Labor.

Enrichment and fortification of foods   A natural development of food industrialization is the enrichment or fortification of foods deficient, or lacking, in certain nutrients. Such policies have implications that should be studied by the Ministries of Health, Agriculture, and Commerce and Trade.

Social and economic implications   The definition of nutritional problems and the establishment of preventive and remedial programs in nutrition may bring about, or call for, changes in attitudes of the population. Some sections of the community may need to change their food habits, perhaps abandoning one palatable food of doubtful nutritional value for another which may be more nutritious but less acceptable. (Changing food habits is the subject of discussion in the next chapter.)

The agricultural production drive may necessitate the establishment of farm cooperatives and whole populations may have to be moved, events that involve considerable social change. The fact that social change is perhaps an inevitable part of a nutrition program should be anticipated and its implications be studied by Ministries of Health, Agriculture, Community Development, Commerce, Labor, Education, and Local Administration. Too little attention has been paid in the past to the side effects of development plans on social behavior and economic status. Some of the results are unpredictable but past experience may allow a better insight into possible repercussions from development programs.[9]

The social and economic status of the community is also affected by the control of food prices or the provision of food *in lieu* of wages. The latter may be desirable provided legislation is available to establish standards for the nutritive value of the foodstuffs. The labor force should be sufficiently organized to insure that the foods are distributed and utilized by the recipients. Innovations such as legislation and distribution of food to labor forces will require the close collaboration of legislators, trade unions, and the management of business enterprises that use migrant labor.

Food consumption   Retail marketing and monitoring of food consumption will probably be one of the principal preoccupations of the central organization. The Ministries of Health and Agriculture will be primarily responsible, but other ministries involved in the marketing and distribution of food may be implicated also.

Financing of programs and services   The central organization will have to determine priorities for executing the program and it will require advice on the financing of programs and services. The Ministry of Finance and the National Planning Board that determines priorities for all government programs would be the most appropriate to fulfill this function.

The prospectus of ministries described above is by no means comprehensive, but it shows the interrelationships of the component agencies and the need for some form of central organization.

Coordination of Ministries]

The next logical step is to study how the various ministries assigned responsibility for the above functions may be coordinated.

This is achieved by the establishment of a body frequently entitled *The National or Central Coordinating Committee on Food and Nutrition* (see Figure 119). Sometimes the body is designated as a *Central Advisory Committee,* but experience shows that advice may not be readily accepted by

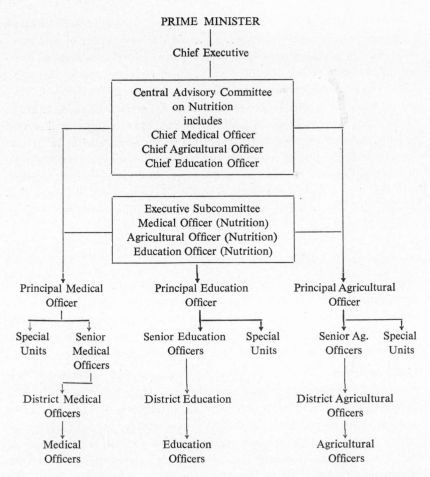

Figure 119   The Central Co-ordinating Committee and its relationships to Regional and Local Administrations

government administrations. The *Central Coordinating Committee* should therefore have executive powers.

Because so many ministries are involved, it is impossible for all the ministries represented on the *Central Coordinating Committee* to be executive. It is also undesirable to assign responsibility to any one ministry because vested interests may influence decisions and executive processes. The executive powers should be assigned therefore, to an executive subcommittee. The ministries most likely to be actively and continuously involved in the development and execution of the nutrition program are the Ministries of Health, Agriculture, and Education. These ministries should form the nucleus of the subcommittee; they may be supplemented by members from other ministries. To avoid undue influence by any particular branch of the government cabinet, the *Central Coordinating Committee* should be responsible only to the Chief Executive, or his deputy.

The rank of the executive subcommittee members is important. They should be in touch with local health personnel, yet they should have access to the office of the most senior administrators in the ministerial civil service. Finally, the staff responsible for executing the program should be able to communicate freely with members of the executive subcommittee without undue hindrance by bureaucratic procedures. Personal experience indicates that the frustrations suffered by executives of nutritional programs and services are often caused by lack of communications with the decision makers in the respective ministries.

Functions of the executive subcommittee

The executive subcommittee should be responsible for the technical administration of the program. The scope of activities of the executives is legion and obviously related to the particular problems of the governments concerned. However, there are some fundamental activities that are common to most nutrition programs and they will be discussed briefly.

Data collection Data pertinent to nutrition should be collected and collated. For example, climatic anomalies should be noted and related to potential food production problems. Food production should be observed and any shortfall in production should be examined for potential nutritional effects. Morbidity data may indicate whether the population is experiencing the clinical effects of deprivation. The rise in case mortality from cummunicable diseases may confirm the onset of overt malnutrition; further confirmation may come from increases in age specific mortality rates.

Qualitative and quantitative changes in food intake may trigger an investigation into the impact of the introduction of a new food of questionable nutritional value. New Labor legislation may have nutritional implications that can be kept under surveillance by examination of sickness reports in industry. The range of possibilities seems limitless but the effectiveness of data collection depends not on quantity, but on making proper inferences. The correct analysis of a situation is enhanced by examining several related sources of information, stressing once again the need for an interdisciplinary approach.

Nutrition services The executive subcommittee should be responsible for the development of nutrition services. These will be in accordance with the priorities fixed by the *Central Coordinating Committee*. Again, the variety of the services is infinite. The actual scope of the services available is described later in this chapter. In broad outline, they include services that exert some surveillance over the nutritional status of the population and detect malnutrition. They may be expected to prevent malnutrition in two ways. First, by direct measures such as increasing food production, by more effective food preservation and processing methods, by more efficient food distribution and marketing, and through welfare services. Secondly, they may help to prevent malnutrition indirectly by improvement of general standards of living, education, better environmental conditions, and control of communicable and parasitic diseases which are synergistic with malnutrition.

Education   The executive subcommittee should be responsible for the improvement of nutrition education offered to professionals and the provision of interdisciplinary education and demonstration programs.

Remedial action   Each country has specific nutrition problems and the executive committee should be responsible for programs and services that bring relief to those already malnourished. For example there may be specific goiter control programs and special medical services established for cases of protein calorie malnutrition, such as the rehabilitation center or the *malward*.

The executive subcommittee may be responsible for dealing with periodic famines or food distribution problems that follow earthquakes and other natural disasters.

The operating level for these functions will be within the framework of the local services of government departments. Sometimes these are relatively simple and arranged on a Provincial or District basis. Figure 119 shows the organizational chart typical of a developing country. Any services involving the Ministry of Health would be executed first through the Provincial Medical Officer and then through the District Medical Officer. In the highly developed countries, there may be State, County, and City administrations that carry a responsibility for providing nutrition services at the local level. They may be funded from Federal, State, County, or local sources thereby complicating the administration, and supervision, of the various projects. The effective provision of nutrition services depends on good administrative organization and technical coordination at all the levels mentioned. The local service has to be made available, it has to be accessible, and it has to be acceptable to the public. Finally, the community must not be neglected or overlooked for little can be achieved without involvement of the people for whom the service is provided.

Further detailed discussion of these various aspects of administration now follows.

The departmental or ministerial representative on the executive sub-committee should be responsible for the coordination of nutrition activities within his or her own ministry. This can best be achieved if a *Nutrition Section* is established within the ministry.

In countries with a simple government structure, this may be a relatively easy task provided there are adequate funds, space, and facilities to support staff and the program. In other countries, it may not be clear which bureau, or division, should be primarily responsible. In some governments, responsibility is given to a physician in charge of maternal and child health services. In others, it is a biochemist working in a food or nutrition laboratory who assumes responsibility. In several countries the responsibility is assigned to divisions offering health education.

A lack of understanding of the true meaning and significance of nutrition by the senior officials who make the decisions, vested interests, or political considerations may make the establishment of a new unit very difficult to achieve. The situation may not be hopeless however, for political influence may change and a bureaucratic stumbling block may retire or be transferred to another department.

The functions of the *Nutrition Unit* are, of course, closely related to the functions of the Central Coordinating Committee, but they focus down on the more detailed aspects of the program. These include data collection, the development of programs and services for the surveillance of nutritional status, the prevention and management of malnutrition, and the education of professionals. Table 82 suggests methods for carrying out the above functions and the units which should collaborate. The organization of effective programs and execution of services calls for personnel of many disciplines, as well as the cooperation of several ministries whose personnel may differ widely in professional education and training. For example, services for the mother and child requires close collaboration between the obstetrician and the obstetrical nurse, the pediatrician, the family doctor, the visiting public health nurse, the nutritionist, the clinic nursing staff, and perhaps the social worker and health and nutrition aide. The reader is invited to consider how the nutrition activities of the various agencies and the programs and services relating to nutrition, may be coordinated in a typical state department of health and the Department of Health Education and Welfare of the United States (see Figure 120 and 121).

It is apparent that the organization of government departments structured like these examples, is not conducive to interunit collaboration. Although

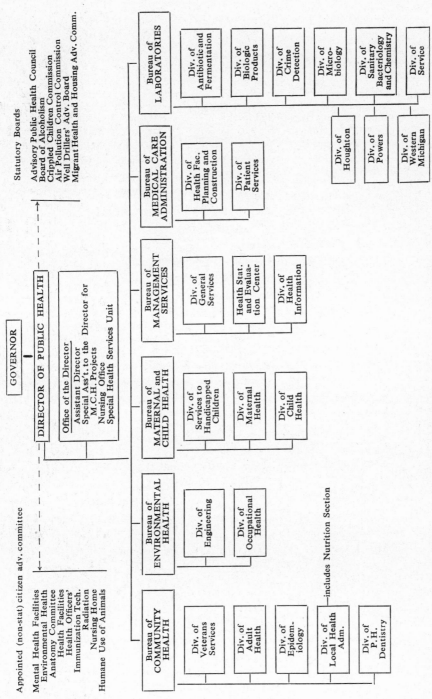

Figure 120 Organizational chart of the State of Michigan, Department of Public Health

DEPARTMENT OF HEALTH, EDUCATION AND WELFARE

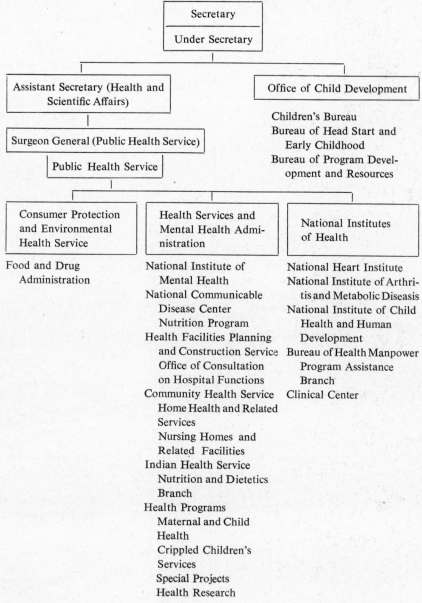

Note: This chart has been simplified for clarity and does not represent the total organization of HEW.

Figure 121   Organization chart of federal agencies offering nutrition programs and services

Table 82 Summary of functions of nutrition unit and collaborating Government units

Function	Method	Collaborating Units In Ministry	Collaborating Units Outside Ministry
Surveillance and detection of malnutrition by:	Vital and Health Statistics	Statistical section, hospital records, reports from health units	Registrar births and deaths
Data collection			Government Statistics Office
	Economic Indices		Government Statistics Office
	Food Balances		Government Statistics Office, Ministry of Agriculture
	Sampling Surveys and "Rapid Surveys"	Nutrition unit, provincial hospitals, health units, pathological laboratories, environmental health units	Agriculture extension Public Schools
	Anthropometry	Nutrition unit, health units	Schools, Preschools, Institutions
	Food Analyses	Food hygiene	Food Laboratories Institutions
Detection and protection of vulnerable groups	Maternal and infant care services	Health clinics, hospital O.P.	Welfare clinics, voluntary organizations
	Preschool child services	Preschool health clinics	Day Care Centers, Kindergarden schools
	School health services	School Health Unit	Public Schools, school nurse service, school feeding programs
	Services for adolescents	Adolescent clinics	Schools, labor and employment advisory centers
	Services for the handicapped	Clinics, hospitals for handicapped	Voluntary organizations, labor and industry, welfare services: institutions
	Services for chronic diseases	Diabetic, renal, cardio-vascular, obesity clinics	Voluntary organization and private foundations

Table 82 (*cont.*)

Function	Method	Collaborating Units	
		In Ministry	Outside Ministry
Detection and protection of vulnerable groups (cont'd)	Geriatric services	Geriatric clinics	Voluntary organizations, welfare services, Meals on Wheels service, community feeding
	Services for the worker	Industrial health	Industrial feeding
Specific preventive programs against:			
P.C.M. chronic malnutrition	Hospital Malwards Rehabilitation Centers	Hospitals Hospital O. P.	Welfare Education, Welfare
	Nutrition Clinics Applied nutrition projects	Rural Health Unit Health	Education, Welfare Agriculture, education, community development, welfare
Goiter	Surveys	Nutrition Unit	Government Statistical Office, Education, Industry, Agriculture
	Iodization of salt		
Anemia	Surveys Drug supplement	Nutrition Unit Maternal and infant care projects	Schools, welfare, voluntary organizations
		School Health Unit Adolescent clinics Chronic disease clinics Geriatric clinics	
	Fortification and enrichment of food	Health Department	Agriculture, food labs, industry
Education and training	Professional and academic	Teaching hospitals, Schools of Nutrition and Dietetics, Nursing schools Laboratories	Universities, Institutions, Teacher training colleges, Laboratories Community development Home economics
	Sub-professionals	Health aide training projects	Home aide and nutrition aide training projects

Table 82 (*cont.*)

Function	Method	Collaborating Units In Ministry	Outside Ministry
Specific preventive programs (cont'd)	Public education	Nutrition and health education projects, Public information unit	Gov't., mass media, radio, T. V. Farmers newspapers, Agriculture extension
General Measures	Improved socio-economic status, Improved health and environ-mental status	Environmental Health Community Mental Health	Agriculture, social welfare, industry, community develop-ment

there is no workable model to copy, or adapt, the organization of the head-quarters of the World Health Organization has many advantages, and tends to encourage collaborative work (see Figure 122).

Broad related areas of operation are brought under the direction of an Assistant Director General. Although there is no clear delineation of re-sponsibilities, the Headquarters administration has assigned these so that their functions fall roughly into five groups:

Administration,

Environmental health, health statistics, editorial and reference services,

Program development coordination and the control of food additives and drugs,

Epidemiology, communicable disease, and biomedical sciences,

Health promotion and protection, education and training, and public health services.

The assignment of responsibility of some of the functions to a particular division is difficult to understand, but it will be seen that most of the disci-plines involved in the detection and surveillance of nutritional status are to be found in the Division of Health Protection and Promotion. The disciplines concerned with the provision of services for the protection of the vulnerable groups are within the Division of Public Health Services while the education and training component of nutrition programs are under the egis of the Division of Education and Training. Most of the nutrition activities can therefore be handled, in theory, under one Assistant Director General. For matters pertaining to Food Control and Environmental Health, there are clear lines of administrative communication laterally through each of the other Assistant Director Generals. Despite some limitations, this type of

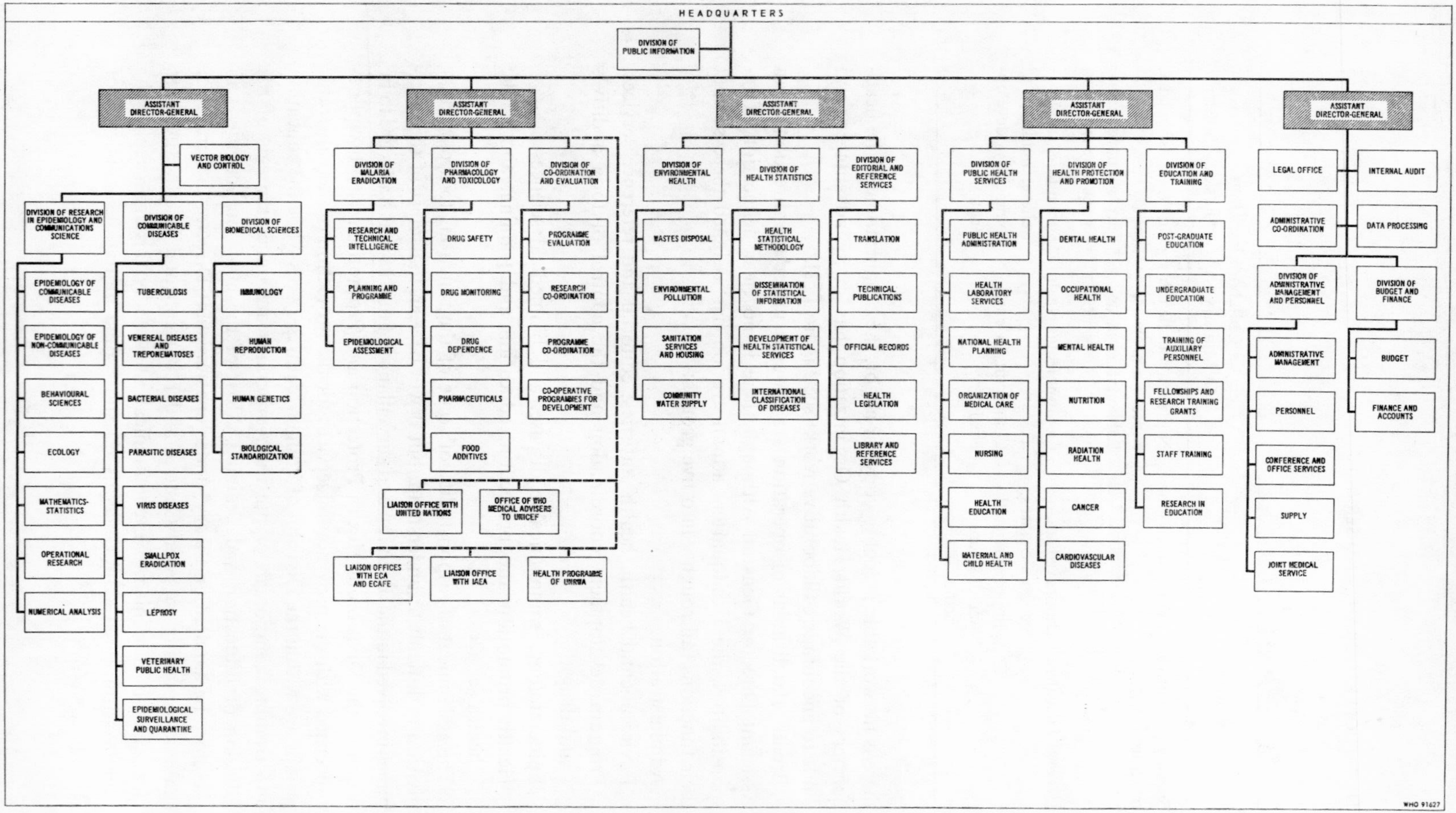

Figure 122   Organizational chart of WHO Headquarters, Geneva (Reproduced from *Official Record 179* (1971)

administrative organization offers many advantages and presents a much better opportunity for a *Nutrition Unit* to function more effectively than the traditional categorized system. While the World Health Organization is commendable from the point of administering nutrition programs, the global organization of nutrition programs presents serious problems. Responsibility for developing programs through the United Nations specialized agencies is divided between the World Health Organization (WHO) and the Food and Agriculture Organization (FAO) and the United Nations Childrens Fund (UNICEF).

On a global basis, there is no equivalent of a *Central Coordinating Committee* and a great deal of the efforts of the specialized agencies are retarded or nullified by "demarcation disputes" relating to responsibilities.[10] For example, the World Health Organization is primarily responsible for health, but if the promotion and protection of health depends on the provision of food then program responsibility is delegated to FAO. If in the course of a school feeding program there is a need to exercise some surveillance over the health of the school children, FAO is unable to do this and must call on WHO. The difficulties are frequently overcome by the collaborative efforts of project staff, particularly in *Applied Nutrition Programs*, which will be described in detail later.

For the proper execution of the functions described on page there has to be an executive machine. Nutrition problems affect the community; therefore, if the programs are to be implemented effectively it is logical to suppose that there should be representation at the community level.

Basic health services, agriculture extension, community development, schools, and local education services may form the executive machinery in the community.

Basic health services

In the simplest situation, the basic health service may be limited to a dispensary that offers first aid and treatment for uncomplicated medical conditions such as coughs and colds, diarrhea and intestinal parasites.

In the next phase of development, delivery of services is through the provision of a *Rural Health Center* or *Rural Health Unit*, and its satellite dispensaries. The Health Center accepts referrals for more serious conditions and may be provided with beds for inpatients and a lying-in ward. Outpatient sessions are held regularly and emphasis is placed on health education including nutrition education.

Special attention is directed towards the mother and the child and it is customary for the midwife, based on the center, to make periodic visits

11*

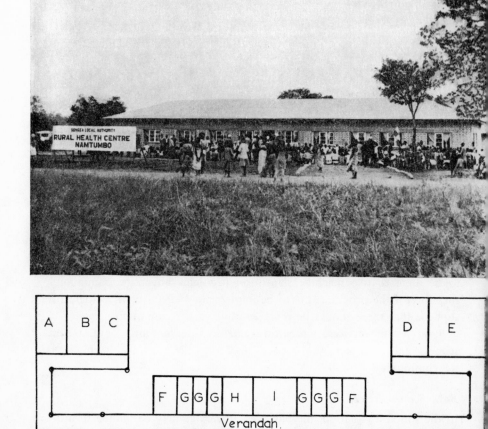

Plate 24   A rural health center in Tanzania. A—kitchen; B—laundry; C—store; D—store; E—labor ward; F—bath; G—WC; H—health inspector; I—lecture room; J—male ward; K—dressings; L—consultations; M—laboratory and dispensary; N—waiting room; O—health nurse; P—female ward; Q—lying-in ward (Photograph by J. R. K. Robson)

to dispensaries where personnel conduct routine prenatal examinations and offer advice. After successful parturition (often in the home under the supervision of the midwife), the mother attends the Well Baby Clinic. This is operated by the public health nurse of the Health Center who also makes regular visits to the dispensary. With more staff facilities and resources, the type of basic rural health service becomes more comprehensive and the reader is referred to other publications on this subject.[11,12,13]

Figure 123 summarizes the function of local basic health services. Cases of malnutrition are first classified; frequently this is based on the Gomez method which uses weight as a criterion.[14] The fallacy of using weights as an index of nutritional status has already been discussed. The possibility of an edematous child being missed is remote and, for practical purposes, the assignment of cases to a first, second, or third degree of malnutrition is to be recommended. The milder cases are referred to supplementary feeding programs, the more severe to rehabilitation centers and the most severe to hospitals. The function and organization of these centers and hospitals will be discussed later. The effectiveness of this system depends on the efficiency of the referral of cases from one unit to another. Experience indicates that this is the weak link in the chain. Referral is not only concerned with the transfer of responsibility from hospital to a rehabilitation unit. It should be concerned also with the referral to other agencies, who may be able to deal with some of the ecological factors that are the root cause of the malnutrition. For example, there may be inadequate, or unsanitary, home conditions promoting the spread of communicable, or parasitic disease. In such circumstances, the referral system should be able to call on the sanitarian for advice. Other members of the family may be vectors of disease; this indicates that a medical examination of the whole family may be required. The mother may be benefit from advice on budgeting from the home economist, or extension worker. The family may be in danger of disintegrating; an event that might be prevented by social workers providing family counselling.

To the complexity that is inherent in public health and nutrition programs, must be added the complications caused by the development of categorical programs. These may include services for the diabetic, the obese, and the handicapped. The lack of flexibility of bureaucratic organization, and deficiencies in interdisciplinary collaboration and coordination, encourages ineffective services. Despite these retarding factors, possibilities for improvement nevertheless exist. However, attention will have to be directed towards a site of operation that has been very much neglected in the past; this is the community. No official can appreciate community

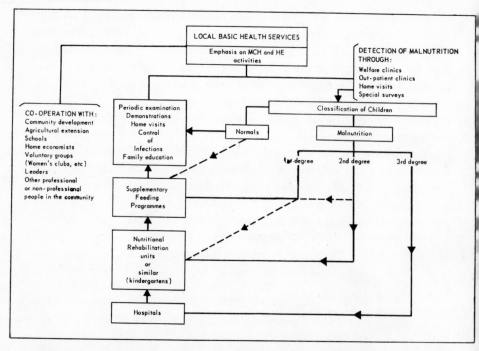

Figure 123   The function of local basic health services (Reproduced from a figure by J. M. Bengoa in *Tropical Pediatrics*, **13**: 175, 1967)

health and nutrition problems as well as the community itself. If the community recognizes the existence of a problem, it is then likely to "feel a need" for programs and services that will bring relief. The delivery of programs and services based on national policies inevitably requires the collaboration of local officials and members of the community. The establishment of a local nutrition committee should be encouraged since so much may be gained through community efforts, and so little without it. With initial guidance from officials, the committee may provide a public forum to inform the community of local or national issues and so help to insure their collaboration in the program. It may be able to coordinate the activities of the various disciplines operating through official agencies, volunteers, and other non-officials in the community. A committee may also be able to exert some political influence at higher government levels.

In advanced countries even more may be achieved. In the USA an opinion is now being expressed that Nutrition Committees are as important today as they were during the second World War when they had a strategic purpose in promoting food production.[15] At that time nutrition committees were functioning in nearly every state; now all but thirty have been disbanded. Their potential usefulness lies in their ability to provide strong leadership. They can act as advisory bodies representing comprehensive resources of expertise, as a clearing house for information, and as a means to initiate programs and services in nutrition. The feeling that the professional is unable to bring about bureaucratic change is widespread. If the prospects for building an organization from the top levels of government downwards are not good, then perhaps the future reorganization of government and the consequent delivery of nutrition services may depend on community organization and its ability to bring pressure to bear from the bottom upwards.

Existing programs and services in nutrition

Irrespective of the lack of coordination, a wide variety of services are provided in the United States. Tables 83 and 84 show Federal, State, local and voluntary agencies which are concerned with the delivery of nutrition services in the United States. In the United States, as in many other countries, the programs and services have developed on an *ad hoc* basis. For the purpose of further discussion the programs and services will be considered under three headings. The first concerns programs and services that provide basic nutritional subsistence; the second discusses consumer protection; and the third will examine programs and services that provide surveillance over nutritional status as well as preventing malnutrition.

Programs that provide basic subsistence

In many parts of the world, attempts are made to insure that each person achieves a basic level of subsistence ensuring adequate nutrition. In the United Kindom, *Social Services* were made available to all after the second World War. The principle law provided insurance benefits during unemployment and after retirement, and financial assistance for individuals in need. For mothers, family allowances of cash were made available in respect of the second and subsequent children.

Other cash allowances and supplementary foods are available to the pregnant mother. *Welfare Foods* are also provided; 82 per cent of the children received free milk and 60 per cent of them received a free mid-day meal in 1963. In Eastern European countries, cash benefits are modest but there are other forms of social assistance including free transportation, special appliances for physical disabilities, and food allowances.[16]

Table 83 National organizations concerned directly, or indirectly with nutrition problems in the U. S. A.

Official

United States Department of Agriculture
    Agricultural Research Service
        Consumer and Food Economics Research Division
    Consumer and Marketing Service
        Food and Nutrition Service
    Cooperative State Research Service
    Economic Research Service
    Federal Extension Service
    Foreign Agricultural Service
Department of Health, Education and Welfare
    Office of Education
    Office of Child Development
    Social and Rehabilitation Service
    Public Health Service
        Consumer Protection and Environmental Health Service
            Food and Drug Administration
        Health Services and Mental Health Administration
            Regional Medical Programs Service
            Indian Health Service
            Community Health Service
            National Communicable Disease Center
        National Institutes of Health
            National Institute of Child Health and Human Development
            Bureau of Health Manpower
        Office of Economic Opportunity
Department of the Interior
    Bureau of Commercial Fisheries
    Bureau of Indian Affairs
Department of State
    Agency for International Development
    Peace Corps

Voluntary

American Red Cross
Foundations:
    National Vitamin Foundation
    Nutrition Foundation, Inc.
Industry-sponsored groups
    for example:
    American Institute of Baking
    National Dairy Council

Table 83 (*cont.*)

Voluntary

National Live Stock and Meat Board
National Research Council—National Academy of Sciences
    Food and Nutrition Board: Committees on food protection, dietary allow-
        ances, amino acids, cereals, fats, infant nutrition, protein malnutrition,
        international nutrition and others
Professional organizations
    for example:
    Americal Dietetic Association
    American Public Health Association
    American Home Economics Association
    American Diabetes Association
    American Heart Association
    Council on Foods and Nutrition, American Medical Association

In the United States, two programs provide basic nutritional subsistence; the first provides food, and the second provides scrip that can be exchanged for food. Examples of the first type are the *Commodities Distribution Program*, and the *School Lunch Program*; the second is represented by the *Food Stamp Program*. All of these programs are administered through the United States Department of Agriculture.

Commodities Distribution Program   The purpose of the Commodities Distribution Program is to provide foods in a way that will not interfere with normal marketing supply and demand. In order to maintain prices, the Department of Agriculture is authorized to purchase food surplus to market requirements. This food may then be donated to schools, to the Bureau of Indian Affairs, and to needy persons residing in institutions, or at home. Commodity foods are processed and packaged; they are delivered free of charge, to State distributing agencies.[17] The Department of Agriculture has established guidelines on eligibility. However, the certification of recipients and the distribution of the food is the responsibility of the cities and counties who choose to participate in the program.

School Lunch Program   The School Lunch Program, established in 1946, has the dual objective of improving the health of children, and encouraging the increased consumption of agricultural commodities. The basic responsibility for the administration of the program is in the hands of State educational agencies. The Secretary of Agriculture is responsible for the establishment of national standards for the program, for maintenance, and general supervision.

Table 84 Organizations at the local and State levels concerned directly or indirectly with nutrition problems

Official

United States Department of Agriculture
    State level
    Country level
Department of Health
    Food sanitation
    Nutrition
    Dietary consultation to institutions
Board of Education
    Health education
    Home economics
    School lunch program
Extension services
Public libraries
State universities

Voluntary

Educational groups
    Private elementary and secondary schools
    Private colleges and universities: home economics, medicine, nursing
    Parent-teachers associations
    Libraries
Social agencies: church and community support
    Children's aid
    Family service
    Salvation Army
    Settlement houses
    Visiting nurse associations
Institutions
    Children's camps, day-care centers
    Hospitals, nursing and convalescent homes
    Correctional institutions
Professional organizations
    State public health associations
    State home economics associations
    State dietetic associations
    State and local medical associations
Civic groups
    Chambers of commerce
    Service organizations
    Women's clubs
Industry sponsored:
    Health centers and hospitals
    Plant cafeterias and restaurants
    Demonstration programs:
        Stores and utility companies

To participate in the National School Lunch Program a school must agree to operate its lunch program on a nonprofit basis and serve lunches that meet the standards established by the Department of Agriculture.

The lunch must be cheap; if children are still unable to pay, they may be given free meals at the discretion of the school authorities.

Table 85 shows the composition of one of the lunches served to each person in the School Lunch Program.

Table 85 Composition of a type (A) school lunch

Food item	Quantity
Fluid whole milk	$1/_2$ pint, served as a beverage
Protein rich food	2 ounces cooked or canned lean meat, fish or poultry
	or
	2 ounces cheese
	or
	1 egg
	or
	$1/_2$ cup cooked dry beans or peas
	or
	4 tablespoons peanut better
	or
	An equivalent of any combination of these in a main dish
Vegetables and fruits	At least $3/_4$ cup, consisting of 2 or more servings. (One serving of full strength juice may be counted as not more than $1/_4$ cup of the requirement)
Bread or its equivalent	Figure 1 slice whole grain or enriched bread
	or
	muffin, corn bread, biscuit or roll made with enriched or whole-grain flour
Butter or fortified margarine	2 teaspoons, used as a spread, as a seasoning or in food preparation

Source: Sandstrom, M. M., School Lunches. Food. The Yearbook of Agriculture. Washington, D. C., 1959.

Under the *Special Milk Program*, the United States Department of Agriculture can subsidize part of the cost of milk provided by schools, nonprofit child-care centers, and summer camps. Schools are also eligible to receive the foods available from the Commodities Distribution Program.

Food Stamp Program The Food Stamp Program is intended to provide a resource that may be used to improve the nutritional status of those in need, and to make more effective use of agricultural productive capacity.[18]

Participants in the program may purchase scrip at a discount price. The coupons are then used in retail stores to purchase food of domestic origin. The eligibility of persons for the program is determined according to state and local welfare standards.

There are certain problems common to the administration of these, and similar programs. Criteria for eligibility to participate, differ according to local welfare standards. Participation can be reduced because of lack of knowledge of the programs, lack of cash to purchase the scrip, and a reluctance to face the challenge of establishing eligibility.

Consumer protection

The programs and services concerned with consumer protection are primarily directed towards the quality of the food that is available for general public consumption. *Wholesomeness* is the concern of the Food Sanitarian and will not be considered here. Once more, the terms used in this aspect of nutrition are used loosely, and sometimes interchanged. Those in most common use are *restoration, enrichment, fortification,* and *supplementation.* *Restoration* is the addition of one or more nutrients to processed foods to restore them to pre-processing (or natural) levels. *Enrichment* is the addition of specific amounts of selected nutrients to a processed food in accordance with official regulations (such as the standard of identity of enriched white bread defined by the U. S. Food and Drug Administration). *Fortification* involves the addition of nutrients to foods and food products that may exceed natural levels. *Supplementation* refers to the addition of nutrients to food.[19] Supplementation may be carried out in a variety of ways and regulations vary from country to country. The following discussion relates to programs in the United States. No enrichment of food is currently required by Federal Law, but, when nutrients are added to food voluntarily, the amounts must conform to standards established by legislation (see Table 86).

Enrichment and fortification of food   Several foods are enriched or fortified; they include table salt, milk, margarine, corn (maize) products, rice, macaroni and other pastas, cereal breakfast foods, wheat bread, and flour.

Table salt has been fortified with potassium iodide since 1924. The program was originally undertaken in an attempt to reduce goiter that was prevalent in the inland, iodine deficient areas of the United States.

Milk. Canned evaporated milk and whole milk has been fortified since 1936 with 400 IU of vitamin D (10 µg of cholecalciferol) per quart of milk Nonfat dried milk can also be fortified with vitamin A or D. Fortification

Table 86 Federal standards for enriched foods
(Minimum and maximum levels in milligrams per pound)

Food	Thiamine	Riboflavin	Niacin	Iron
Bread, rolls, and other baked foods	1.1–1.8	0.7–1.6	10.0–15.0	8.0–12.5
*Flour	2.0–2.5	1.2–1.5	16.0–20.0	13.0–16.5
†Farina	2.0–2.5	1.2–1.5	16.0–20.0	13.0–
‡Macaroni, noodle, paste products	4.0–5.0	1.7–2.2	27.0–34.0	13.0–16.5
Corn meal and grits	2.0–3.0	1.2–1.8	16.0–24.0	13.0–26.0
Rice	2.0–4.0	1.2–2.4	16.0–32.0	13.0–26.0

* Calcium enrichment is also required for self-rising flour.

† A maxium level of iron enrichment for farina has not been established.

‡ Levels of enrichment allow for 30–50 per cent losses in preparation.

was intended to prevent rickets; undoubtedly it has been successful. Margarine, the substitute for dairy butter, is fortified with vitamins A and D.

Corn (or maize) products. The Food and Nutrition Board of the National Research Council has recommended that maize products be enriched with thiamine, niacin, and iron, in those areas where maize meal and *grits* form a substantial part of the diet. Some, but not all of the states where maize is consumed, have adopted laws controlling enrichment.

Rice. If rice is enriched, it must contain thiamine, riboflavin, niacin, and iron. In Puerto Rico all white rice must be enriched.

Pastas. Macaroni, spaghetti, vermicelli, pastina, and noodles are prepared from wheat flour. Most of these products are boiled in water which is then discarded. Because of the inevitable losses of vitamins in doing this, the level of enrichment is higher than other products. Pastas are enriched with thiamine, riboflavin, niacin, and iron. Some products also include added calcium and vitamin D.

Cereal breakfast foods. There are no standards for the enrichment of ready-to-eat breakfast foods but most manufacturers have added nutrients to their products voluntarily. Farinas, finely ground cereal meal, used for the preparation of infant foods and breakfast cereals must comply with government definitions and standards, however.

Wheat, bread, and flour The voluntary enrichment of bread and flour became compulsory during the second World War. After the cessation of hostilities, enrichment became statutory once more. Approximately 30 states have adopted enrichment laws. In these states bread is either made from enriched flour or, enrichment wafers containing thiamine, riboflavin, niacin, and iron, are added during the mixing of the dough.

In the United States, the enrichment of white flour and bread has been based on public health objectives. The consumption of six slices of bread in the daily diet will supply sufficient amounts of thiamine, riboflavin, niacin, and iron to prevent deficiencies of these nutrients. Enrichment has improved nutritional status without changing food habits. The enrichment policy was based on the food habits of 30 years ago. Food habits have changed since then; this may indicate a need for a review of original policies. Formerly most of the flour was made into bread; since that time there has been a decrease in consumption of white flour. This has been balanced by an increase in consumption of purchased sweet baked goods such as cakes, pies, doughnuts, and cookies. Because few of these latter products are enriched, a continuation in this trend would remove much of the value of the present enrichment program. The risk of inadequate thiamine intakes could be avoided by establishing enrichment standards for mixes, cakes, cookies and other bakery products.[20] Breakfast cereal consumption is increasing; in view of the fact that there are no standards governing levels of enrichment in these foods, it is difficult to estimate what the average contribution of breakfast cereals is to the total consumption of thiamine, riboflavin, niacin, and iron. The implications for the future intake of these nutrients is also in doubt.

Other countries around the world also have programs for the enrichment and fortification of foods. The latest enrichment regulations in England are mandatory. Minimum amounts of thiamine, niacin, and iron must be added to all flours, with the exception of whole meal wheat flour; this must also contain calcium. In the Phillipines, the staple food, rice, is enriched with thiamine, niacin, and iron. In Denmark, all white flour, farina and semolina must be enriched with thiamine, riboflavin, iron, and calcium carbonate. The levels of the added nutrients are higher in Denmark than in any other country practicing enrichment. In Canada, the program of enrichment has been voluntary (except in Newfoundland), however it is estimated that about 90 per cent of all the commercially-made white bread in Canada is enriched.

In Australia the addition of nutrients to white bread is statutory and is on a similar scale to that used in the USA. Iodine enrichment including the addition of iodine to bread is used as a public health measure in many goitrous areas of Australia.

Restoration of nutrients is important for food products whose nutrients are either destroyed or extracted during processing or storage. The nutrients concerned may be restored to their naturally occurring levels, or even higher.

In infant foods, foods for the elderly, and food products designed for weight control, many nutrients need to be supplied in a single serving. Sometimes these products supply all needed nutrients or they may be designed to complement the nutrients found in milk. In order to insure that the serving meets recommended allowances the products are often fortified with nutrients far above natural levels.

Nutrients are sometimes added to products for non-nutritional reasons. Ascorbic acid and vitamin E, for example, are sometimes added to foods to prevent the oxidation of other unstable compounds.

The problems of protein inadequacy in developing countries have directed attention towards the fortification or supplementation of indigenous diets that are based on poor quality protein. It has even been suggested that the deficiencies of protein, vitamins and minerals would be relieved by mandatory supplementation of each cereal.[21] This suggestion is unduly optimistic and fails to take into account many practical difficulties that exist in developing countries. The lack of road and rail communications, inadequate marketing, distributing, and storage facilities would not allow national fortification and supplementation of cereals. Much of the food at the subsistence level is home produced and it is unlikely that premixes of nutrients could be made available to the individual farmer. In addition to this, the cost of supplementation has been estimated to increase costs of the food budget by 3 or 4 per cent.[22] This represents an increase that would be beyond the budgetary capabilities of many wage earners in developing countries.

In addition to these mundane problems, the effect on metabolism of fortifying cereals with amino acids has also to be given serious consideration. Most of present day knowledge of amino acid balance and requirements has been acquired through experiments on man and other animals. There is evidence that the quantitative and qualitative amino acid requirements may differ at the low levels of protein intake that are usual in the problem areas of the world. The infant or child who has been receiving a protein deficient diet may have difficulty in catabolizing excess essential amino acids. The accumulation of essential amino acids in the blood may lead to a reduction in food intake. The metabolism of non-essential amino acids is unaffected. It is also known that an excess of a single amino acid can limit growth and may even be toxic. In the well fed, an excess of an amino acid such as lysine would cause little side effects but in protein deficient children an excess of this amino acid could antagonize the utilization of arginine by the body. There is also a risk that the provision of lysine to a diet of poor quality may mean that another amino acid becomes the limiting factor; if this amino acid is not readily available growth may still be retarded. It should also be remembered that the provision of a supplement may stimulate growth. This phenomenon may increase the requirement for other nutrients such as vitamin A. If the intake of this or other nutrients was marginal before supplementation the intervention of growth may precipitate a deficiency state. Finally, it should be remembered that if the calorie intake of the population is inadequate the amino acids in the fortified cereal may be used for energy production instead of growth.

The quality of food offered to the consumer may depend on other non-food materials that are added to enhance keeping qualities or appearance. These materials are known as additives, as they have important health implications they will be discussed in some detail.

Food additives   An additive has been defined by the Food Protection Committee of the Food and Nutrition Board of the National Research Council of the United States, as "a substance or mixture of substances, other than a basic foodstuff, which is present in a food as a result of any aspect of production, processing, storage, or packaging. The term does not include chance contaminants". There are two broad types of additives. The first is the *intentional* additive; these are substances added on purpose to perform specific functions, such as, preserving the quality of the food, or improving its nutritive value. Salt and spices are long used additives, both enhance the flavor of the food, in addition salt is used as a preservative. The second type of additive is the incidental additive; these are substances that may have no function in the final food product. They may however, become part of a food product during production, processing, storage, or packaging. Agricultural chemicals applied to crops and carried over to processed foods are common incidental additives. The total number of known additives exceeds 20,000[23] and they have 45 different uses.[24] These are summarized in Table 87. Additives that improve the nutritive value of certain foods include iodides in salt, vitamins in fortified milk, margarine, bread, wheat flour, corn flour, and rice.

The flavor of food is enhanced by many diverse additives including spices, essential oils, and aromatic chemicals such as the artificial flavorings, pineapple and cherry. Many of the last category are used to insure that the flavors of seasonal foods are available all year. Other substances are flavor enhancers; they do not add flavor themselves, but they bring out the natural flavor in food. *Monosodium glutamate* is one of the best known flavor enhancers.

Table 87 Summary of function of food additives

Function	Example
Improve nutritive value	iodine in salt, enriched bread, rice
Enhance flavor	salt, sugar, spices, monosodium glutamate
Maintain appearance, palatability and wholesomeness	
Antioxidants	ascorbic acid, BHA, BHT
Preservatives, antimycotics	salt, benzoic, acid, calcium proprionate oxytetracycline
Improve and maintain consistency	
Emulsifiers	cholic acid, ox bile extract
Stabilizers and thickeners	agar-agar, ammonium citrate
Control acidity and alkalinity	sodium bicarbonate, acetic acid
Leavening agents	sodium bicarbonate, potassium acid tartrate
Coloring agents	carotenes, cochineal, saffron, caramel, synthetic colors
Improve baking qualities	mono- and di-glyerides, sodium stearyl fumarate
Sequestration of undesirable chemicals	citric acid, EDTA
Preserving moisture	sorbitol, glycerol
Prevent caking	calcium silicate, silica gel
Promote firmness in fruits and vegetables	calcium chloride, calcium citrate
Provide non-nutritive sweetening	saccharine, cyclamates

Antioxidants prevent spoilage in color, or flavor, caused by exposure of food to the oxygen in air. In the home, darkening of fresh fruits is prevented by dipping them in lemon, orange, or pineapple juice. These juices contain vitamin C, an antioxidant that is used in great quantities commercially. Rancidity in fats is due also to oxidation, and can be prevented by a number of chemical antioxidants that have a greater affinity for oxygen than the food material.

Molds, bacteria, and yeast, cause food spoilage; their growth can be prevented or inhibited. Salt and sugar have fulfilled this function for many years. Antibiotics are now used to retard spoilage of poultry and some fish products.

Additives can be used also to give, or maintain, desired texture and thickness in food. Some are emulsifiers which facilitate mixing of two or more immiscible liquids such as salad oil and vinegar. In addition to facilitating the mixture they also help to maintain the state of emulsions. Emulsifiers are widely used in the baking industry. Stabilizers and thickeners maintain the physical characteristics of food and help to maintain flavor.

Buffering agents facilitate some food processes by adjusting the pH of the material. Acidifying agents add a "tartness" or acid taste to foods. Leavening agents facilitate baking and make the baked product light in texture. Coloring agents have an obvious function; formerly all colors were natural in origin, now 90 per cent of coloring materials are synthetic. They have the advantage of being more uniform, more stable, and cheaper than natural pigments. A high proportion of the coloring materials formerly in wide-spread usage have been prohibited as additives because of the possibility that they may be carcinogenic.

Maturing and bleaching agents are used widely in the baking industry to facilitate the production of bread and bakery products. They insure that the food is devoid of natural pigments that might spoil the appearance. They also modify the characteristics of the wheat gluten thereby ensuring that successive batches of bread are consistent in texture.

The amounts in additives in food vary, some of the quantities are minute but this does not exclude them from being potentially dangerous. Much more biochemical information is required concerning additives and their metabolism. Although animal experimentation may show that some additives are harmless, much less is known of their effects on the health of man. Human experiments are usually conducted on a small scale and the long term effects can only be the subject of speculation. There is also the possibility that harmless agents may be converted to dangerous substances, by the body. For example the intestinal flora may be able to convert *cyclamates* to cyclohexamine, a compound toxic to humans. Very little is known of the interactions, or interrelationships between *intentional* and *incidental* additives.

Recently, concern has been expressed over the safety of *monosodium glutamate* and *cyclamates*. *Monosodium glutamate* (*MSG*) is one of the most ubiquitous of all food additives. Commercially prepared frozen meat or fish, dry soup mixes and many canned goods contain *MSG*. It is used to intensify the flavors of soups, chowders, canned meats, stews, sea foods, and cheese spreads. One of the chief active ingredients of soy sauce is *MSG*. Its mode of action is not understood. Formerly it was believed that its main property was due to its own meat flavor. This has, however, been shown to be an artifact. It is possible that it may increase the sensitivity of the taste buds or stimulate the formation of saliva. *MSG* injected or fed into the stomachs of infant animals has been shown to cause lesions in the hypothalamus. The lesions have been associated with disorders of regulation of food intake and disturbed endocrine function. Other research has established the sensitivity of infant nervous tissue to *MSG*. In early infancy the ability to detoxify glutamic acid to glutamine is limited; this facility increases progressively during infancy. In view of the possible danger from the ingestion of *MSG* early in life, some major food manufacturers no longer include this additive in infant foods.

Cyclamates are artificial sweeteners. It has been found that they are capable of inducing mutations in chick embryo cells. In high concentrations, cyclamates have also caused bladder tumors in rats. Legislation in the United States demands that any food additive must be removed from the market if it has been shown to cause cancer when fed to man or animals. In the USA cyclamates are only available now by medical prescription. The effect of cyclamates in rats cannot be directly related to man and there is no indication that bladder cancer is increasing to any significant degree. *Saccharin*, the other non-nutritive sweetener is still recognized as safe for use in foods.

Incidental additives such as pesticides, and mercury, may prove to be more dangerous than the *intentional* additives. The former may be even more dangerous to populations consuming poor quality diets. In animal experiments it has been found that Endrin was most toxic in rats, fed from weaning, on a protein deficient diet.[25]

National agencies are usually responsible for drafting legislation controlling food quality. However, the enforcement of the legislation is becoming more and more difficult as the number of products made available for consumption increases. Convenience foods and packaged foods have facilitated the concealment of inferior products or materials that are not listed on labels. Because of these problems the Food and Drug Administration of the Department of Health, Education and Welfare in the United States has adopted a legal labelling standard for certain nutrients. A selected list of vitamins and minerals are included in the *Minimum Daily Requirements*. Special dietary foods, such as infant formulae, and weight reduction formulae, must show the percentage of the *Minimum Daily Requirements* that would be satisfied by the consumption of a stated amount of the food product (see page 315). The Federal Food, Drug and Cosmetic Act as written in 1938 and subsequently amended, forms the basis for regulation of food additives in the United States.

Many countries have also adopted standards of uniform quality. In the United States, a system of grading exists for more than 100 foods including meat, dairy, and poultry products, fruit, vegetables, and grain. The regulations are reinforced by an inspection program; however, this is only applied to products shipped from state to state. It is possible under existing laws for products within states to reach the market without inspection.

The inspection and grading of products does not, furthermore, guarantee that the product will reach the consumer in the same condition as when it was graded.

Surveillance and preventive services

The function of nutrition services may be summarized into four main categories. These are, surveillance of nutritional status, promotion of proper nutrition, prevention of malnutrition, and the rehabilitation and treatment of malnourished patients. Table 88 summarizes the method and place of operation for surveillance and prevention of malnutrition.

An ideal service would fulfill all of these functions throughout the life cycle. This is not feasible in practice. Services have been developing piece-meal and there is inevitably some overlapping of function on the one hand, while one particular need may not be met by any of the services.

Surveillance This is not limited to surveillance of nutritional status, for it is important that a watchful eye be kept on total health. A regular routine physical examination should provide some reassurance that the child is maintaining a life relatively free from sickness. A child constantly affected

Table 88 Summary of method and place of operation for surveillance and prevention of malnutrition

Action	Method	Place
Surveillance	Clinical and routine health examination Regular measurement of height, weight, skinfolds Biochemical assessment of nutrients in blood and urine Biophysical assessment including radiographs of hand and wrist Diet history	In the physicians office, the hospital and clinic and the home In outpatient clinics, Well Child Conferences. Special projects including Day Care Centers, Creches, Preschool and School Clinics
Prevention	Health promotion Prevention of infection Supplementary feeding Mineral and vitamin supplementation Education	In the physicians office, the hospital and clinic and the home Outpatient clinics, special projects Special clinics, special projects and school

by coughs, or colds, or diarrhea, is nutritionally *at risk*. Many mothers consider repeated and frequent attacks of gastro-intestinal disturbances as part of the normal pattern of infancy. Surveillance should include, therefore, questioning at regular intervals to ascertain the infants' morbidity experience. In East Africa, where urinary *schistosomiasis* is common, the passage of blood in the urine of children is considered quite normal and

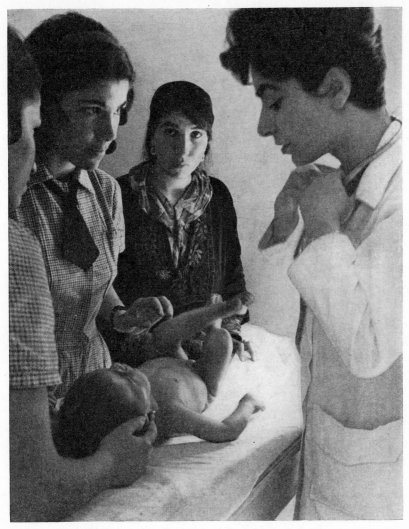

Plate 25   Surveillance of child health in Jordan. A regular routine physical examination provides reassurance that the child is maintaining a life free of sickness (WHO photograph)

mothers frequently seek advice because their children have not yet experienced hematuria.

Depending on the scope of the services, it may be possible to conduct biochemical tests during the course of routine examinations. Iron status may be determined either by measurement of serum transferrin (which also gives information on protein status), by hemoglobin estimation, or by the simple method of measuring the specific gravity of blood as described in Chapter 3. In highly industrialized countries the urine may be tested for the presence of phenylalanine.[26,27]

If growth and development is monitored, delays in maintaining "normal" progress should be detected. Measurement of height, weight, chest, and head circumference, and skinfold thickness should be carried out regularly throughout the growing period. The recording of the data on suitable charts will allow progress, and changes in velocity of growth, to be assessed. Children who are underweight, overweight, underheight, or who have abnormal skinfold thicknesses, can be detected by these relatively simple procedures. If the facilities are available, it is sound practice to x-ray the hands and wrists to determine whether there is a delay in ossification. When disturbances in health, growth, or abnormalities in body tissues, tissue fluids, or radiographs are detected, the infant or child should be referred for further examination and study. This should include an appraisal of his food habits and dietary intake.

The services providing surveillance need not be very sophisticated, nor do they always require highly educated or trained staff. If accurate data are to be obtained, care is required, but routine weighing and measuring is within the capabilities of voluntary workers, nurses, schoolteachers, or health aides. Questioning on morbidity experience, and the collection of dietary data, can be carried out by suitably trained sub-professionals. Surveillance should be feasible within most health services and should be incorporated in them whenever possible.

The infant and child welfare clinic is one of the most common services provided by rural dispensaries or health centers. They provide an ideal situation for surveillance. In sophisticated health systems the Maternal and Infant Care Projects of urban ghettos and the Well Child Conference of affluent suburban areas can be used as a base of operation.

Professional staff may resist the introduction of new services because of a fear that it may add to the work load. Experience shows that the provision of nutrition surveillance may actually bring benefits. An ongoing experiment is examining the feasibility and advantages of providing surveillance over the nutritional status of infants in Michigan. Several benefits

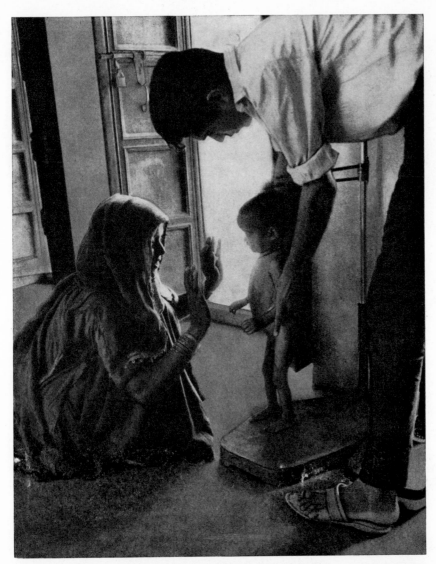

Plate 26 Measuring weight and height in India (WHO photograph by Claude Huber)

which had not been anticipated by the Local Health Department are emerging. For example, by simple measurements it has been established that more than 16 per cent of the "apparently healthy, well fed children" who are using the clinic, are below the third percentile of nationally used standards for height and weight. This important observation had not been previously noted. The measurement of infants is not only screening out those who may have nutritional problems but also infants and children with medical and emotional problems. The technique seems to be a useful way to detect infants with disturbances in health that might otherwise have passed unnoticed.

Following-up infants in the home provides an opportunity to inquire into the health of other members of the household. In the Michigan study, the problems of the family seems to be establishing a closer working relationship between the nutritionist, the nurse, and the family physician.

Surveillance should not be restricted to the normal child. Children in the category *Failure to Thrive* are another important group needing continuous surveillance (see page 418). These children have already experienced growth retardation because of emotional deprivation. The conditions which originally led to the growth retardation may have been only temporarily alleviated. The mother should be encouraged to bring her child for regular appraisal after discharge from medical care.

In many health programs there is a lack of services for the preschool child, and the *secotrant* (the child in his second year of life) who is especially *at risk*. The practice of measuring infants while they attend the clinics may habituate the mother to continue attending throughout the second year of life, and perhaps even longer.

In general, however, the provision of surveillance over the preschool child must be achieved through special preschool programs including *day care centers* or *creches*. They usually require special funding, many require a high degree of organization, and trained staff. Their function is described in further detail later in this chapter.

In countries with few resources, *day care centers* and *creches* can be organized with local facilities. The former may be centered on the activities of women's clubs, perhaps operating from a village community center. The supervision of the *day care center* may be the responsibility of the health nurse or the community development worker. Many of these centers exist in impoverished communities. Usually the mothers take turns to look after their infants and children.

Creches may be established in industrial organizations as an incentive for mothers to continue to work. The *creches* provide a similar opportunity for some simple surveillance procedures.

The supervising nurse of the school clinic may monitor growth and development, but in many schools, routine weighing and measuring is the responsibility of the teacher. A regular record of growth may be continued throughout school life, providing continuous information on growth achievement, and giving warning of interruption or abnormality. The adolescent period is one of some concern, for it is a time when weight problems become apparent and when food fads and emotional disturbances are liable to interfere with the food and nutrient intake. Consequently, obesity, growth failure, retarded mental development, skin blemishes, and pregnancy, are the most frequent reasons for teenagers seeking nutrition counselling.[28] The specific problems of growth failure may be real, or apparent, because of the delays in the onset of menarche. It has already been pointed out in Chapter 5 that there is a wide variation in the time of onset of puberty. An apparent failure to grow may be caused by a delay in the adolescent growth spurt. Surveillance and reassurance of the young adolescent may be the only treatment required, but it may prevent an interlude of emotional disturbance.

The downward trend in the percentage of unmarried mothers in the USA has been accompanied by a rise in the number of unwed mothers under the age of 18 years.[29] This has resulted in special programs and services being developed for teenagers. The service may provide education as a substitute for the formal variety that is lost when the young mother has to leave school, as well as informal maternity and nutrition education. This may be supplemented by offering general counselling advice on grooming, and the provision of opportunities to learn skills that may be useful for the mother when she has to seek employment. There is evidence that such services have reduced perinatal mortality and second unwed pregnancy. Services in pregnancy is the subject of a separate discussion later in this chapter.

The infant born of the adolescent mother frequently falls into the category of the *low birth weight* baby whose problems have been discussed in Chapter 5 (see page 401). The onus of surveillance of *low birth weight* babies first falls on the hospital or nursing home staff who deliver the baby. Hypoglycenia is a danger facing all twins and babies who are less than the 25th percentile for weight on appropriate standards, and they should have their blood glucose levels monitored after delivery.

The surveillance of the growth and development of the infants should continue while the child remains in the hospital and there should be an immediate referral of the baby after discharge to programs that will continue to keep a close watch on his future progress. Surveillance of nutritional status of adult populations is virtually non-existent. From morbidity and mortality data, certain disease states such as cardio-vascular disease, diabetes, and obesity, have obvious importance. Because of their relationship with food and nutrition, some surveillance is exerted within categorical programs. Screening for diabetes may reveal overweight persons; routine medical, examinations for life insurance may reveal high serum lipid levels. Liver function may be tested in programs and services for alcoholics and drug addicts.

For most populations in the world, health surveillance of the adult is neglected, yet as the breadwinner and the one responsible for the welfare of the family, the health and nutrition status of the head of the household is vitally important. The value of surveillance has been recognized by some industrial organizations. Executives who are at risk to cardio-vascular disease, because of their sedentary and dietary habits, and exposure to stress, are submitted to regular examination. This service should be extended throughout industry for cardio-vascular disease is not exclusive to the executive.[30] Surveillance of the aged presents many practical problems. The aged are readily "lost" in modern cities and remote rural areas so the population at risk may not be known. Because of physical disabilities, impoverishment, or lack of transportation, the elderly tend to be immobile. Consequently regular medical checks in the physicians office, or in the agency clinic may be impossible.

Social workers and public health nurses have access to the homes of the aged, and they can supervise their well being. Communication between professionals (or their aides) of the various disciplines visiting the home, is important. There are times following bereavement, discharge from hospital, and financial worries, when the elderly are particularly at risk. It is important that these events be made known to the private physician, the social worker, and the public health nurse.

Promotion of health and prevention of malnutrition   In theory this may be considered separately from surveillance but usually promotion of proper nutrition is integrated into programs providing surveillance. The promotion of health is also very much related to the protection of health. For example, the immunization programs of health agencies protect the child against smallpox, poliomyelitis, measles, diphtheria, tetanus, whooping cough, and typhoid. In many countries vaccination against tuberculosis with BCG is an important factor in protecting the health of the young child.

The provision of vaccines and other immunizing agents is often the incentive that brings mothers and their infants to the clinic. It is unfortunate that health departments tend to become so preoccupied with this service that other aspects of the clinic operation are often neglected. When the infant and child completes its schedule of inocculations the child frequently "drops out" of the clinic routine.

Not all diseases can be prevented; gastro-intestinal and upper respiratory infections will continue to add stress to the growing child. Parasites invade the body and tissues of young children; only rarely can they be prevented by direct means. The health programs and services which help to control these diseases must be considered part of the armamentarium of services for the promotion of better nutrition.

Malaria control measures and environmental sanitation that reduces the incidence of enteric disease and parasites should not function in isolation. The nutritionist should see if existing programs can be used and exploited in the interests of nutrition. Conversely, where there are nutritional problems, the nutritionist should try to stimulate fellow professionals to improve communicable disease control, community water supplies, and environmental health.

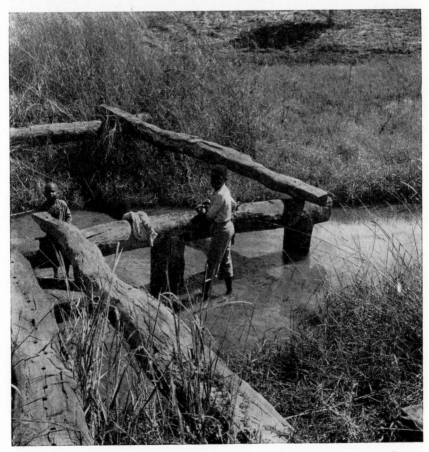

Plate 27   Environmental health. This stream in Tanzania was the source of many cases of *bilharzia*. A nutrition program should take note of *foci* of infections and infestations and attempts should be made to reduce the incidence of communicable disease (Photograph by J. R. K. Robson)

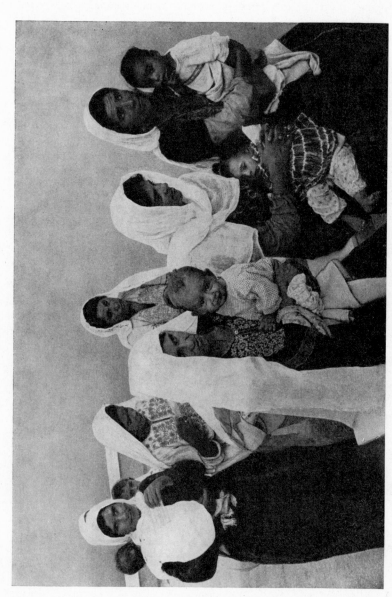

Plate 28   Education in a Well Baby Clinic in Jordan. Mothers are given advice on infant feeding, weaning techniques, and child care (WHO photograph)

Education is an important factor in promoting health. The clinic is an excellent medium for providing information, and educating mothers on child care, infant feeding practices, and home-craft. During school years and in adolescence, education may be an important factor in teaching the child the basic concepts of a proper and adequate diet. Nutrition education may be offered formally in the school curriculum, or it may be part of the clinic activity. It should be noted however, that the provision of educational facilities, and opportunities to learn proper eating habits, does not necessarily mean that diet habits will change.

One of the more obvious ways to promote health and promote better nutrition is to provide meals. If this is not possible, snacks should be provided. The importance of food in insuring attendance at school and promoting alertness has not been fully evaluated but studies of the effects of school snacks on a school population in Africa were encouraging.[31] Children receiving a variety of protein rich foods including dried skim milk, peanut flour, soya bean flour, and meat powder experienced greater growth than a control group. The groups that received the snacks were reported as being more attentive and regular in attendance than the controls.

School meals may help to "condition" a child to certain eating habits. The role of school meals and similar programs in bringing about change in dietary habits is discussed in the next chapter. The village *day care center* and the *creche* also provide a medium for the provision of food and education. The provision of food on a regular basis to very young children not only helps to maintain and improve nutritional status, but other beneficial health habits may also be learned. For example, in the *Bayambang Applied Nutrition Project* in the Philippines, which is described in detail later, the habit of washing hands before a meal was introduced. The adoption of this simple practice could lead to improvement in standards of hygiene that may help to reduce the incidence of cholera, enteric disease, amebiasis or the non-specific gastro-intestinal disorders, which are a feature of life in Filipino *barrios*.

The provision of meals may not be feasible; as an alternative, diet supplementation of whole communities has been attempted. In Peru, a study was made of the effect of giving additional food for a period of five years to a disadvantaged community whose children were experiencing poor growth and a high infant and child mortality. There was a decline in mortality experience but growth performance was no better than that observed in two control populations.[32] The problem of controlling experiments such as this is extremely difficult and the true effects of the supplementation may have been masked. The investigators conclude that the supplements

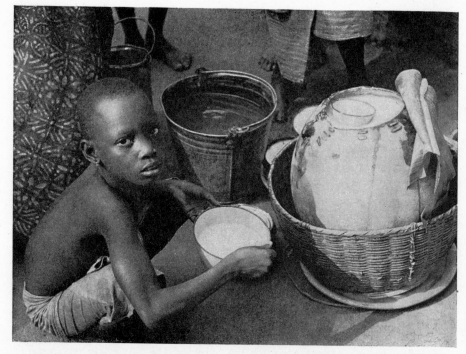

Plate 29   Breakfast for a schoolboy in Dahomey. Many schoolchildren may have nothing more than a bowl of cassava for breakfast and this may have to suffice until they return home in the late afternoon (Photograph by Professor H. A. P. C. Oomen)

may displace other food. If this occurring, the supplementation would only have a beneficial effect if the displaced foods are of lesser biological value.

Supplementary foods may be offered to mothers on behalf of their infants. The dried skim milk supplied by UNICEF has served an invaluable role in many parts of the world. The problems of distributing the milk in many developing countries is formidable, and only partly solved by issuing it though child welfare clinics. There is no doubt that the milk can provide a great incentive to attendance. In a clinic in Songea District in Tanganyika, the weekly attendance at the Well Baby Clinic rose from an average of 8 infants per day to over 60 per day after UNICEF milk became available. There is no guarantee that the milk is ever given to the infant, but this risk should not deter milk distribution. One of the problems frequently encountered in programs providing dried skim milk is the poor, and inappropriate advice that may be offered with the milk; possibly the worst is to advise that the milk be reconstituted with water. Not only does this result in a milk unpalatable to most tastes but it unfortunately also carried with it

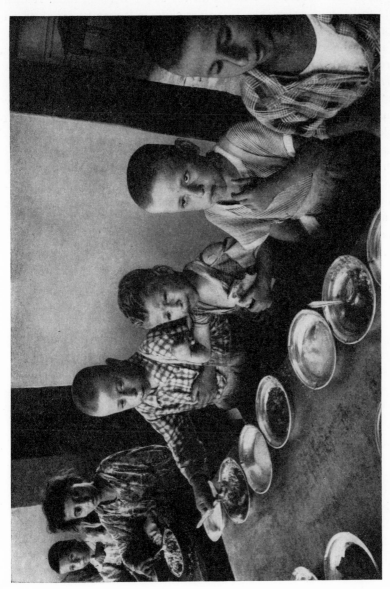

Plate 30 School feeding in Jordan. School meals are important, a substantial meal like this provides good quality protein and adequate calories; the latter ensures that the protein is available for growth (WHO photograph)

the risks of gastro-enteritis through the use of contaminated water supplies. The milk is usually most needed where the standards of hygiene are low. Dried skim milk should be mixed with the staple weaning food. It then appears to be quite acceptable. For older children it may be sprinkled on rice, or mixed in with relishes stews, or gruels.

Nutrient supplements may also be offered by health agencies. In infancy the provision of iron may be important where iron deficiency anemia is prevalent. However, where the need is greatest, the regular issue of vitamins is frequently not feasible. Where supplements are not essential, the early introduction and continued ingestion of vitamins by infants, in the form of tablets and pills, is unjustifiable.

There is no doubt that in certain areas vitamin deficiencies are dangerous and prevalent and they should be prevented if possible. Rickets can be controlled by the use of food products fortified with vitamin D. This practice is not without its health hazards. The dangers of over-ingestion of the nutrient have already been mentioned (see page 24).

Vitamin A deficiency can be eliminated with economic growth and education, an event well exemplified by Japan whose population formerly experienced serious deficiencies of this vitamin. Not all countries can enjoy such meteoric changes in fortune. In the meantime, attempts to increase the consumption of green leafy vegetables by infants and children and the use of red palm oil for cooking should be continued. These preventive efforts should be reinforced by providing vitamin A as a diet supplement. The provision of codliver oil or sharkliver oil is effective but costly. In rural areas where transportation is a problem, it may be impractical. The fortification of dried skim milk with vitamin A has been prescribed but doubts have been expressed concerning absorption of the vitamin from a vehicle which is almost fat free. In a study in Brazil, it was concluded that vitamin A is absorbed and that the fortified dried skim milk does help to maintain serum vitamin A levels.[33]

The body usually treats large doses of vitamin A as a poison but recent field studies have indicated that hepatic storage of vitamin A can be achieved. An oil-soluble preparation of vitamin A administered orally, as a single dose of 50 mg can maintain serum levels for six months afterward.[34,35] Protection may also be obtained by administering red palm oil to children as a "vitamin medicine".[36]

Provided the mothers diet is good, the breastfed baby can derive enough vitamin C from the mothers milk. Cows milk is a less reliable source; with the current trends towards formula feeding, vitamin C supplementation may be advisable in infancy.

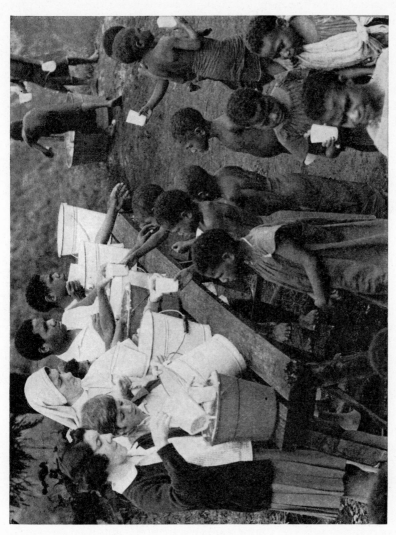

Plate 31 Supplementary feeding. If a whole meal cannot be provided, a snack may help to maintain growth and health. These children in New Guinea are being given milk at their Mission School (Photograph by Professor H. A. P. C. Oomen)

Hemorrhagic disease of the newborn caused by vitamin K deficiency may be prevented by giving this vitamin to the newly born baby. Usually this is a responsibility of the obstetrical services.

Endemic goiter is preventable; the role of iodization of salt in achieving this objective for whole populations is discussed later. However, iodized salt may not be available for distribution on a national scale. In such circumstances, iodized oil given by injection may be an effective goiter control measure.[37] The method is cheap and its effects may last as long as four years. The injections can be given to all ages of the population using local health services. In a few cases there may be side effects and for this reason programs should only be carried out under medical supervision. This should include surveillance to see if signs of *hyperthyroidism* are developing. The regime involves the intramuscular injection of iodate in oil and it may be given to the entire population and repeated after two years.

In more affluent countries specific health programs with nutritional components have been established.

The *Head Start Program* in the United States is for the benefit of the child in poverty who is recognized as having health problems. Identification of the problem alone is insufficient, and the services provided by *Head Start* projects involves education of children, families and even professionals. When attempts are made to provide new and innovative services for the child in poverty, deficiencies in existing services become very apparent. This points out the value of examining the resources of health agencies continually.

Children and Youth projects are intended to provide a continuation of the services offered by the *Maternal and Infant Care* projects. Like the *Head Start Program*, it is primarily meant for deprived children for whom comprehensive care is available if the medical, health, dental, and psychological evaluation of the child shows need. Appropriate treatment on an individual basis is provided either through the project or through related services. Innovative components are encouraged, one example being a program designed to reduce the incidence of lead poisoning in the urban ghetto.

Nutrition education is considered important and may be offered to parents as well as youth. Nutritionists in *Head Start* and *Children and Youth* projects evaluate diets and counsel families on normal nutrition, budgeting, and the fulfillment of diet prescriptions for specific feeding or nutritional problems. The success or failure of these projects lies in inter-disciplinary collaboration, good referral and the presence of other health, medical, and dental services, which are accessible and acceptable to the family.

Special nutrition programs and services

Special problems arise in both the developing and the highly industrialized countries. Sometimes the problems are peculiar to one or the other. For example, special services for large numbers of cases of protein calorie malnutrition are unlikely to be required in highly industrialized countries. Conversely, programs for the prevention of cardio-vascular disease would not have a high priority in the health plans of a developing country. However, in both deprived and affluent societies the nutritional status of the pregnant mother is vital to the well being of the future infant population. In most countries, Maternal and Child Health Programs are the backbone of health programs. There is, however, an unfortunate tendency to separate the health care for the mother and her child into two components. The first part is concerned with the pregnancy and its outcome. This tends to be looked on from the point of view of the obstetrician who is concerned with achieving the full term delivery of a healthy baby. Although it cannot be denied that the prenatal period is of vital concern to the nutritionist nutrition counselling by a suitably qualified person may not be available at many ante-natal clinics. The Well Baby Clinic does not begin to look after the infant for some time after delivery. This important period when the infant is virtually without surveillance is a time of critical growth. The "service gap" could be bridged by providing a special service for the pregnant and lactating mother and her child.

Other specialized services will be considered under the headings of obesity, prevention of cardio-vascular disease, and nutrition services for the aged. The main need in developing countries is for services to deal with the problem of protein calorie malnutrition. This will be discussed under the headings of rehabilitation, special hospital wards (*malwards*) for the treatment of malnutrition, and *Applied Nutrition Programs*.

Nutrition services for the pregnant and lactating mother

In developing countries, maternal mortality rates may be high because of poor environmental conditions, lack of proper maternal and health care, and poor diets. With improved conditions, maternal mortality rates fall but the fetal and infant mortality rates remain sensitive indicators of reproductive efficiency. The significance of these rates has been discussed in Chapter 5. Low birth weight, perinatal handicaps, and failure of the infant to grow and thrive are other indicators of inadequate reproductive performance.

13*

Low Birth Weight   Pregnancy is influenced by many interrelated factors (see Figure 124). Some of these may interact adversely and result in low birth weight. A low socio-economic status for example, may be associated with poor nutrition. The effects of the poor nutrition may be aggravated by infections which are liable to be more frequent in the deprived sections of the population. The impoverished may have unsafe water supplies, inadequate sanitation, and a squalid environment. Lack of health care may allow chronic diseases, malaria, and other parasitic disease to continue to drain the health of the women of reproductive age. Poor socio-economic conditions may be associated with pregnancy at an earlier age. This is important because the risk of low birth weight is much higher in the biologically immature mother under seventeen years of age. The first born, and the fifth and subsequent child, are also special risks. Poor nutrition may have a direct effect on fetal immaturity and may also prevent females from reaching their full genetic potential. Shortness of stature itself, is associated with low birth weight and high perinatal mortality (see Table 89).

Low birth weight is not confined to the poorer nations of the world. In the United States, teenage pregnancy in unwed girls is increasing and

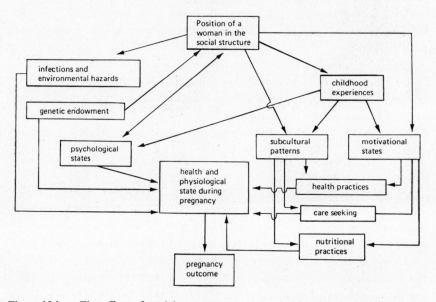

Figure 124   The effect of social structure on women's physiological state and on pregnancy outcome (Original figure by Dr. J. R. Udrey, reproduced from *Maternal Nutrition and the Course of Pregnancy, 1970* by permission of the National Academy of Sciences)

there are urban ghettos and depressed rural areas with poor socio-economic and health conditions. In the affluent sections of North America, the diet of many adolescents is poor because of the habit of snacking, and consuming carbonated beverages. In addition, there are other adolescents who intentionally eat a restricted diet in order to preserve the slimness of their figures.

Table 89 Incidences of low birth weight, and perinatal mortality in Scottish (Aberdeen) and Chinese (Hong Kong) primiparae, by maternal stature

Height (in)	Birth weight under 2500 g %		Perinatal deaths per 1000	
	Aberdeen	Hong Kong	Aberdeen	Hong Kong
Under 57	16.3	19.3	40.7	19.2
57–58		11.6		
59–60	10.3	6.6	28.6	17.3
61–62	6.9	6.7	25.7	
63–64	6.2	5.7	24.4	14.4
65 and over	3.7			

Source: Thomson, A. M., Billewicz, W. Z., *Proc. Nutr. Soc.* **22**: 55 1963.

Weight gain is an inevitable part of pregnancy. However, excessive weight gain leads to concern for health, consequently recommendations have been made on what should be considered a desirable weight increase during pregnancy.

It was formerly believed that protein provided the main contribution towards weight gain. It is now realized that it is fat, and not protein, that is stored during pregnancy. The normal range of weight gain is difficult to define because of the wide variations observed (see Table 90). In industrialized countries, a gain of 10–12 kg appears to be representative of gains in healthy women on a "normal" (unrestricted) intake of food. Excessive weight gain may be due to a large fetus, abnormal amounts of *liquor amnii*, fat, or fluid.

Pregnancy is accompanied by a considerable increase in total body water; excessive amounts may become apparent as edema. There is divided opinion on the significance of clinical edema. It has been considered a dangerous sign, but it has also been noted in many women who have produced healthy babies after an uncomplicated gestation and parturition.

Table 90 Average gain in body weight, measured from first trimester of pregnancy

Author	Subjects	Average gain (kg)
Kerwin, 1926 (USA)	Mostly "labouring class"	7.5 (range 2.7 to 17.3)
Plass and Yoakum, 1929 (USA)	Private patients, normal pregnancy	17.0
Lawson, 1934 (USA)	Normal private patients in "comfortable circumstances"	10.9 (range —5.4to+20.0)
Pugliatti, 1937 (Italy)	Abnormalities excluded	10.4
Stander and Pastore, 1940 (USA)	Normal healthy pregnancies	12.8
Kuo, 1941 (China)	Selected for normality	Primigravidae 10.6 Multigravidae 9.7
Kerr, 1943 (USA)	Normal healthy pregnancies (women who lost weight excluded)	10.4
Tompkins and Wiehl, 1951 (USA)	Not stated	10.9
Humphreys, 1954 (UK)	Normal healthy pregnancies	Primigravidae 11.7 (S.D.3.8) Multigravidae 10.7 (S.D.3.8)
Thomson and Billewicz, 1957 (UK)	Primigravidae with normal blood pressure	11.4
Ihrman, 1960 (Sweden)	Unselected hospital patients	10.2
Venkatachalam, Shankar and Gopalan, 1960 (India)	Poor-class women employed in tea plantation	Primigravidae 5.4 ± 0.76 Multigravidae 6.2 ± 0.44

Source: Nutrition in Pregnancy and Lactation
World Health Organization. Technical Report Series No. 302. p. 20.

Generalized edema has been related to *toxemia* of pregnancy and it may be an exaggerated and pathological manifestation of normal edema. The electrolyte balance in pregnancy is not fully understood and probably will remain so until further study is made of the role of sodium in the development of edema and toxemia. The term toxemia does not correctly describe the condition for it is not caused by an accumulation of toxic products in the body, but is applied to all hypertensive disorders of pregnancy. Criteria and reporting procedures for toxemia vary widely from country to country, and even within countries, hence comparative studies are often impossible. The extent of toxemia in various parts of the world is unknown. In the United States, toxemia has been associated with low income groups and is common in non-whites.[38] However, this latter association is probably not related to any biological differences in the races, but to deprivation of health and medical care for non-whites.

The low incidence of *toxemia* in the Far East and Central Africa has been attributed to racial and dietary differences. Climate and geography can be excluded, because in Fiji, Trinidad, and Panama, where different races live in the same environment, the prevalence of toxemia varies in the racial groups.

Any pre-existing abnormality of the vascular, metabolic, or endocrine systems predisposes to toxemia. It is therefore common in *diabetes mellitus*, hypertension, and where there are abnormalities in the products of conception. It is also associated with physiological immaturity and multiple pregnancy. Severe emotional stress, poverty, and nutritional deprivation are also probable etiological factors but surprisingly, obesity is not necessarily a predisposing factor.

A relationship between calorie and protein intake and toxemia has been assumed, but there is little definite evidence of this relationship. In Europe during the first World War, there was a decrease in the incidence of severe toxemia which was believed to be related to the dietary restrictions imposed on the populations at that time. Calorie restriction became a universally accepted therapeutic procedure in toxemia. Both high and low protein intakes have been incriminated as the cause of toxemia. The high intakes were thought to place a load on kidney function but this theory has been discounted.

Hypoproteinemia has also been blamed, but in India no significant difference was observed in the ratios of urea nitrogen to creatine excretion in toxemia and normal women. This tends to exclude disordered protein metabolism as an etiological factor.[39] Vitamin B_6 deficiency has also been blamed as a causal factor because of reports that the early symptoms of toxemia (nausea and vomiting) were relieved with the administration of pyridoxine hydrochloride. There is little to support this hypothesis, moreover dietary deficiency of this vitamin is virtually unknown.

Sodium has been incriminated in the etiology of *eclampsia*, which is the severe manifestation of toxemia. During pregnancy the blood volume normally increases. Since the concentration of sodium in the plasma of pregnant women is normal, it follows that there must have been retention of sodium. This is believed to be achieved by changes in the endocrine control of renal excretion. There is no apparent increase in the proportion of sodium in the plasma in *eclampsia* for the sodium levels are within normal limits in this disease. It has been noted, however, that after delivery, *eclamptic* patients may lose large quantities of sodium in their urine.

Because of this last observation, pregnant women have been advised to restrict their intake of sodium; there is no physiological or definite pathological reason to justify this. In sodium restriction there may be an excessive stress placed on the system responsible for the hormonal control of sodium retention. In rats, exhaustion of hormonal secretory cells of the juxta-glomerular apparatus of the kidney tubule and the adrenal cortex, have been noted. It is believed that similar harm may result in humans subjected to sodium restriction.[40]

There is an increase in the blood volume during pregnancy. The increase in the volume of cells is proportionately less however, so there is an apparent hemodilution. In addition to this there is frequently a real decrease in hemoglobin levels that may adversely affect the health of the mother.

One of the physiological changes in pregnancy is the increase in hemopoesis which increases nutritional requirements. The iron for erythropoiesis may be derived from the stores. Usually the stores are inadequate to meet the demand and the balance has to be drawn from the normal food intake, but in the indigent the diet is often inadequate. The dietary deficiencies may be compensated by an increase in utilization of iron. The high prevalence of anemia indicates that the supply still does not meet the demand and supplementation with iron may be necessary in deprived populations.

Folate deficiency is common in developing countries; in the highly industrialized areas of the world, megaloblastic anemia is usually confined to the poorer sections of the population. Anemia may also follow acute blood loss, infections, or parasitic infestations including malaria and hookworm.

Osteomalacia caused by an inadequate intake of vitamin D is a hazard of pregnancy in developing countries. In all parts of the world including affluent countries, if pregnancy intervenes before the cessation of bone growth there may be inhibition of development of the bony skeleton. The effect of malnutrition on the fetus has been discussed in Chapter 5. It must be stressed that the differential growth of the fetal tissues calls for highly specific nutrient requirements. If the mother cannot meet these needs, then fetal abnormalities may occur. Because of the special needs for protein and amino acids, it is obvious that calorie inadequacy may be especially dangerous.

The care of the pregnant and lactating mother   Dietary management must be related to the nutrient needs in the prenatal and postnatal period. Services should provide counselling, and surveillance of health, throughout gestation, and lactation.

Prenatal care In addition to normal obstetrical surveillance, the food habits, dietary patterns, and food intake of the mother should be ascertained. Any dietary deficiencies should be noted and the patient advised on how the nutrient intake may be improved.

Weight gain should be monitored, and the skinfold thickness measured at regular intervals to see if the normal pattern of fat deposition is being followed. Skinfold thicknesses normally increase up to 30 weeks of pregnancy, and decrease between 38 weeks and the end of pregnancy. The increase in skinfolds is greater in the underweight than the overweight.[41]

Biochemical determinations may be used to evaluate iron and folate status. While depletion of iron stores takes time and precedes clinical anemia, the serum folate levels are affected very early in dietary deficiency. Even though excessive weight gain may be occurring, dietary restriction is contra-indicated during pregnancy, and weight control should be deferred until after delivery.

The adolescent requires particular care; she should preferably attend special clinics for young mothers where she may be offered counselling and education appropriate to her needs.

In developing countries where protein intakes are marginal, the provision of dried skim milk to pregnant women is fully justified. Not only does it provide much needed nutrients, but it provides an incentive to the mother to return for regular examinations.

In the more affluent societies, vitamin and mineral supplements should not be used as a palliative for bad food habits. Where iron and folate deficiency have been found, there is no doubt that therapy, including supplementary iron and folate, should be given. It is assumed that the provision of mineral and vitamin supplements will be effective, but little is known of the value of routine supplementation of iron. During a recent experiment in Britain, 32 per cent of a group of women failed to take iron tablets given them at an ante-natal clinic.[42]

Lactation The lactating mother and infant are one biological organism. The diets of both are regulated in early infancy through the maternal metabolism, since the milk supply of the mother appears to be adjusted to the needs of her infant. Later, the infant receives an additional independent food source of its own. Diet regimes for mothers do not take this supplementation into account, and the recommended intakes of nutrients, may be quite unrealistic.

With respect to calorie intakes, it has been suggested recently that the energy cost of lactation is much less than anticipated. It is now believed that the efficiency of conversion of energy from the mother to the milk is in the region of 90 per cent. This would mean that an intake of an additional 600 calories would support lactation.[43] Successful lactation can be achieved on less than the recommended allowances for other nutrients which indicates that they are all too liberal. Health care should insure that lactation is established and maintained. Lactation is taken very much for granted, but little is known of how many women are able to produce adequate milk for feeding their infants. The trend towards formula feeding may be hiding sections of the population who have failed to lactate. An increase in the incidence of failed lactation could have serious consequences in populations dependent on breast feeding. The incidence of failed lactation is virtually unknown, but in Iran, it was found to be much more common than anticipated (see Table 91).

Table 91   Failed lactation in urban and rural areas of Iran

Location	Numbers	Lactation Failure	
		Complete	Incomplete
		%	%
Rasht City	35	3	6
Rural Villages	68	15	6

Source. Dr. G. R.Wadsworth and H. Emami, Food and Nutrition Institute, Teheran, Iran.

In India, failure to breast feed is almost unknown in the poorest social classes but in the affluent and educated sections only about 20 per cent of women breast feed infants. This proportion is similar to that observed in highly industrialized countries.

A complete inability to secrete milk may be caused by severe undernutrition in childhood which has led to impaired development of the secondary sexual characteristics and inadequate mammary tissue. The growth and development of the mammary tissue during fetal life is known to be affected by sex hormones but there is little information on the effects of nutrient deprivation.

Nutrient deprivation of the mother may interfere with the development of the mammary bud in the second month of fetal life, or subsequently in the third, fourth, and fifth month of fetal life when the primitive milk forming apparatus is undergoing differentiation. If there is interference

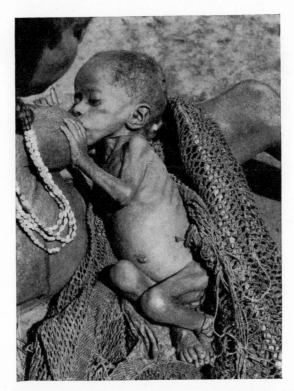

Plate 32   Failed lactation in this New Guinea mother is the cause of this marasmic baby (Photograph by Professor H. A. P. C. Oomen)

with cellular hypoplasia, there may be a decrease in the numbers of elementary milk glands.[44] If there is inadequacy in development of primitive breast tissue then maternal deprivation may have an indirect effect on the second generation. The affected fetus may successfully complete gestation and grow to maturity and become pregnant. Her failure to lactate places her offspring *at risk* to protein calorie malnutrition. If this should occur it would have been caused by events which took place 15–20 years previously.

It has been suggested that failed lactation may be a genetic adaptation and the consequence of disuse of the mammary gland for several generations. The repeated emptying of the breast helps lactation while accumulation of milk suppresses milk production, consequently the abandonment of demand feeding may encourage failure of lactation.

The continuation of breast feeding is vital to the health of many infant populations; for this important reason alone there is justification to promote better lactation performance. Counseling on lactation should start early in pregnancy to insure that mechanical problems due to inverted nipples do not prevent suckling at a later date. Teaching hygiene may reduce the risk of breast abscesses. Mothers should be counseled also on a proper food and fluid intake for it has been noted that drinking water beyond the natural inclination, suppresses lactation.

In developing countries, mothers should be encouraged to consume a wide variety of foods to decrease the risks of producing milk that is lacking thiamine or vitamin C.

The prevention and control and treatment of obesity

The basic cause of obesity is an intake of calories in excess of energy expenditure. The reasons for this energy imbalance are many and varied (see Chapter 1).

One cause is genetic in origin; weight control in these cases may prove to be almost impossible. There are other causes of obesity however, that are preventable. There is evidence that some obese persons are fat because they have an excess of fat cells; this excess of fat cells being produced during early life.[45] It is possible that early weight control may help to break the cycle of events that turns a fat baby into a fat child who becomes a fat adult who produces fat babies. Infants who suffer from hypertrophic obesity (obesity associated with enlargement of adipose tissue cells), rather than the hypoplastic obesity described above, may be conditioned to overeating. This could be the result of being fed excessive amounts of cow's milk in early infancy. This type of obesity should also be subject to control. Similarly, obesity should be anticipated in children with handicapping conditions that limit their activity.

There are other causes of obesity which may be preventable in theory but practical prevention and control may be very difficult. Obesity caused by emotional disturbances and obesity related to cultural habits and practices are examples of such cases.

The estimation of calorie intakes and the regular measurement of body weight and length should help to detect the child who is becoming fat. Similar surveillance should be continued during school life. Other individuals *at risk* such as the disabled, physically and mentally handicapped, should be identified and placed under surveillance. This may be done in institutions, in weight control programs in school, in adolescent clinics, or in specialized agency programs for the obese. In the older age groups those *at risk* include the returning war veteran and the retiring athlete who may have become conditioned to a high calorie intake through years of high energy expenditure. It will also include the worker recently promoted from an active job to a sedentary executive position.

The detection of cases and the treatment of obesity should be part of an overall program for weight control. There is little point in identifying victims of overweight if they cannot be referred for the specialized treatment which obesity demands. Because of the complexity of the etiology of obesity, it is obvious that the treatment must be planned for each individual. There should be ample trained staff to determine the causation of overweight and to insure that the recommended therapy is feasible and acceptable to the patient.

A negative calorie balance may be achieved in three ways; first by reducing the calorie intake and keeping activity constant, second by increasing the activity and keeping the intake of food constant, or finally by increasing activity and decreasing intake. In addition to diet control and increased activity, other measures must be included in any weight control program. These include the management of environmental stress that encourages overeating, education and psychological support.

Diet control   It has been recommended that the diet should contain 14 per cent protein and 30 per cent fat. The latter should contain a minimal amount of unsaturated fats. The remainder of the diet should be carbohydrate with the total intake of sucrose reduced.[46]

The high protein content is advised because it not only provides a feeling of satiety, but a portion of the caloric content is used in its own metabolism (see page 227). The low sucrose and saturated fat intake is prescribed because of the possible relationship between these nutrients, high serum lipid levels, and the risk of heart disease; a risk already present in overweight patients.

In obese infants and growing children, the restriction of diet should be viewed with caution. It has been shown that not only is the energy expenditure reduced but the intake of many obese babies is also less than normal children. Care should be taken to insure that reduction of the food intake does not result in growth failure.

Starvation may be used as a temporary measure in grossly obese adult patients who have not responded to other forms of therapy. It should only be undertaken in a hospital under close medical supervision. Metabolic responses and electrolyte changes, should be assessed regularly. In starvation, the body is in negative potassium balance; in addition the effect of therapeutic agents may be exaggerated. Obese patients with cardiac dysfunction may be endangered by the electrolyte disturbances and perhaps by the effects of diuretics and drugs controlling the heart beat. Despite these hazards, starvation is an effective method of treating obesity and should be safe for 7 to 14 days. Weight loss in this period may be from 18 to 36 pounds. In prolonged fasting of more than 40 days, electrolyte disorders, protein deficiency, anemia, and malabsorption of vitamin B_{12} have been encountered.[47]

Low calorie formula diets are available; these have limited use for they do nothing about retraining food habits. They have a value in the early part of therapy when the patient is being instructed on proper diet therapy. In general, the monotony of low calone diets does not allow them to be used for protracted periods.

Anorexigenic agents may be given to allay hunger pangs and are best used when hunger becomes a distressing feature of the reducing diet. The effective duration of treatment with drugs is from four to six weeks. There are varying individual responses to appetite depressant drugs. They should only be given under medical supervision; they should never be given to patients with defective heart function.

Adding bulk to food decreases its caloric density without reducing the volume or satiety value of the food, however, palatability may be impaired. There is a tendency for starchy foods to be avoided in weight control regimes so that bulked foods may not be acceptable to the prescribed regime. A reduction in palatability would also be likely to cause rejection of bulked foods by the obese who are more sensitive to the taste of food. Elimination of salt from the diet is generally not recommended in weight reduction programs unless clinically indicated. Mild salt restriction tends to minimize fluid retention and may be effective in controlling any tendency to hypertension.

Other measures, including thyroid and growth hormone preparations, diuretics, and surgery to bypass the small intestine, have had little success in weight control programs.

Exercise Increasing the expenditure of energy may prove to be difficult; the very obese may have difficulty in movement and their cardio-vascular systems may not be able to tolerate more than the gentlest of exercise. It should also be remembered that the obese expend less energy than persons of normal body composition. It has been shown that a 250 pound man walking 1.5 m.p.h. expends 5.34 kilocalories per minute whereas a 150 pound man carrying a 100 pound load expends 5.75 kilocalories per minute walking at the same pace.[48] Obese children can exercise with a considerable economy of effort.

Management of Environmental stress   As the intake of food is governed to some extent by environmental stress, it follows that therapy should remove as much of this stress as possible.[49]

It has been shown that hunger in obese persons is less related to gastric motility than in normal persons. The obese tend to respond more to cues related to external events; for example, obese patients will respond to time shown on a clock even though the clock may be running "fast" or "slow" compared with the correct time.[50]

When cues are absent as they would be on religious fasting days, obese subjects are more likely to observe the restrictions than the normal individual.[51] Fear has less influence, and taste more influence, on food intake in the obese than the non-obese. It would seem reasonable to assume that the identification of cues which either stimulate or depress eating might be used in weight control programs. A series of procedures may be drafted for an individual which might be used to reinforce eating habits that discourage weight gain and weaken habits that encourage weight gain (see Table 92).

Education   Patients must understand that the basic cause of obesity is a long-standing faulty balance between dietary intake and energy expenditure. They must realize that permanent adjustments in the pattern of living may be necessary and that a certain amount of self control and effort will be called for, if the program is to be successful. The patient should know the calorie content of foods in their various portion sizes, and the effect of food preparation on its calorie content.

Psychological support   Regardless of the type of regime suggested, the physician, dietitian, or nutrition consultant has to show genuine interest and sympathy towards the patient. Threatening the patient with the dire results of overweight should not be part of treatment and they should not be given unrealistic prospects of favorable results. The complexity of obesity, and its treatment, means that well organized staff and facilities are required. Usually the onus for providing these services fall on institutions and the local health authority.

One of the features of weight control programs is the use of patients of voluntary and private organizations typified by *Weight Watchers* and *TOPS* (*Take Off Pounds Sensibly*) which use dietary counselling, exercise, and group therapy as a basis for their activities.

Results from weight control programs are generally poor and in one study it was estimated that only 8 per cent of obese patients seen in a nutrition clinic actually maintained a satisfactory weight.[52]

Table 92 Sample procedures used to strengthen appropriate eating and to weaken inappropriate eating

Cue elimination	Cue suppresion	Cue strengthening
Eat in one room only Do nothing while eating Make available proper foods only: a) shop from a list; b) shop only after full meal Clear dishes directly into garbage Allow children to take own sweets	Have company while eating Prepare and serve small quantities only Eat slowly Save one item from meal to eat later If high-calorie foods are eaten, they must require preparation	Keep food, weight chart Use food exchange diet Allow extra money for proper foods Experiment with attractive preparation of diet foods Keep available pictures of desired clothes, list of desirable activities

Reduce strength of undesirable responses   Increase strength of desirable responses

Swallow food already in mouth before adding more Eat with utensils Drink as little as possible during meals	Introduce planned delays during meal Chew food slowly, thoroughly Concentrate on what is being eaten

Provide decelerating consequences   Provide accelerating consequences

Develop means for display of calorie value of food eaten daily, weight changes Arrange to have deviations from program ignored by others except for professionals Arrange to have overeater re-read program when items have not been followed and to write techniques which might have succeeded	Develop means for display of caloric value of food eaten daily, weight changes Develop means of providing social feedback for all success by: a) family; b) friends; c) co-workers; d) other weight losers; Program material and/or social consequences to follow: a) the attainment of weight-loss subgoals; b) completion of specific daily behavioral control objectives

Success can be predicted to some extent; poorer results have been noted in persons over fifty compared with those under fifty years old. Similarly, being from a lower socio-economic group, having a body weight 60 per cent more than normal weight, being divorced or separated, is associated with failure rather than success.[53]

With the recent introduction of behavioral control of obesity there has been renewed hope for the obese.[54,55]

Nutrition services for the aged

The elderly are particularly at risk to malnutrition. This may be largely attributed to the food intake of the elderly being very much dependent on the sociology of eating.[56] Loneliness, eating alone, poor cooking facilities, and financial worries lead to depression, apathy, and lack of initiative. In such circumstances it is virtually impossible to purchase, prepare, and consume a proper and adequate diet.

Aging is frequently accompanied by a breakdown in health. Physical disabilities such as arthritis, strokes, or dental problems may be responsible for formidable feeding difficulties. It is known that one of the problems of aging is the gradual loss of cells. It is generally assumed that the nutrient requirements for the aged are greater because of physiological inefficiency including enzyme deficiencies and malabsorption. There is however, surprisingly little evidence that physiological inefficiency is due to the aging process alone.[57] The determination of nutrient requirements is difficult. Pathological conditions frequently exist in old age; they either interfere with function or create additional nutritional demands on the body. Chronic infections in the gastro-intestinal tract, for example, may do both. The failure to meet the extra demands may mean a further deterioration in health and the establishment of a vicious circle.

The prevalence of malnutrition in the elderly population is not easy to determine. The dietary intake is not a reliable index of nutritional status. Clinical signs may not be helpful either, since it is sometimes difficult to decide whether a sign, such as edema, is the result of hypoproteinemia or whether it is the result of vascular disorders. The nutrient levels in tissue fluids may suggest depletion, but this may not be confirmed by disturbance in function or clinical examination.

In developing countries, little is known of nutrition problems in the aged. In the highly industrialized countries, adequate information is also lacking but serious vitamin deficiencies are probably rare. There is evidence of low intakes of certain nutrients and from clinical observations it is apparent that the elderly are liable to anemia, and deficiencies of ascorbic acid, folic acid, thiamine, and vitamin D. Surprisingly, overweight tends to be a problem rather than underweight.

Iron deficiency anemia is more common in females than males but both sexes are affected by folic acid deficiency; this latter disease is considered to be the most common vitamin deficiency in Britain. Osteoporosis, which may be as much due to a lack of solar radiation as vitamin D inadequacy, is a common debilitating disease in the United States.

The prevention of malnutrition in the elderly may use several approaches. First, measures are needed which will help to promote general health; this will help to reduce the incidence of disabling conditions that may lead to secondary nutrient deficiencies. Secondly, there must be the provision of social and welfare services that will give financial assistance where necessary and enable the elderly to purchase an adequate diet. They may need help in household management, a service offered by the *Home Help Service* in the United Kingdom and the *Homemaker Service* in the United States. Services such as these are probably the greatest contribution to the prevention of malnutrition among the elderly. However, the service tends to be limited by financial stringency and recruitment of suitably motivated staff. In Newcastle on Tyne in England, the total number of hours of help available to each old person was 4.9 per week. This is, of course inadequate for shopping, cooking, and domestic work. Only 1.1 per cent of the population over 65 have a meal cooked by a home help.[58]

There should also be an available source of supplementary nutrients and food and even whole meals. Vitamin and mineral supplements can be provided without difficulty in institutions. For the old person living in isolation, the provision of nutrients may require attendance at clinics or visits to the office of private physicians. The availability of special geriatric clinics and home visiting services would facilitate the provision of a supplementary food and nutrition program.

Meals can be provided at *day centers* for the elderly. In Detroit, Michigan, the Department of Parks and Recreation provide catered lunches for the elderly. Transportation is provided; this is a necessity for programs whose participants may be partially or wholly disabled, or who live some distance from the facility. The *day centers* also provide opportunities for education and weight control instruction.[59]

The food intake of married couples is found to be far superior to that of single persons living alone. Whenever an old person is able to eat with a family or friends, and share communal life for part of the day, the food intake increases. The mobile elderly can take advantage of *luncheon clubs* which provide a hot meal and some companionship. For these to make a real contribution to the nutritional status of the elderly, clubs should be open at least four or five times a week. *Luncheon clubs* also provide an opportunity for surveillance since non-attendance can be noted and followed-up by a home visit.

The *Meals on Wheels* service provided by local authorities and a womens voluntary organization in England provides a hot meal every day for those who can neither shop nor cook and who may not be able to travel to a *day center*. The effectiveness of *Meals on Wheels* depends on the service being provided frequently, and regularly. A meal given less than three or four times a week cannot maintain adequate nutrition. The meals may be prepared and distributed by a central kitchen, school kitchen, residential home or by institutions. Day to day distribution is fraught with hazards when the weather is inclement. There are also problems of acceptability because of fussiness and the variability of food preferences in the aged. Nutrient losses in the cooking procedures or during delivery of the food may be considerable.

In most countries services for the aged are badly needed and sadly lacking. Most health departments have many unfulfilled obligations to the senior citizens and their nutritional status.

Diet in the prevention of cardiovascular disease

In the United States, the United Kingdom, and Sweden, arteriosclerotic heart disease is the commonest cause of death. In the discussion of Chapter 3 it was pointed out there was no direct cause and effect relationship between the diet, high blood lipid levels, atherosclerosis, and coronary heart disease. The contribution of stress, smoking, and sedentary life cannot be assessed. In preventing cardiovascular disease, diet and other environmental factors have to be considered. Health education and health services should encourage the cessation of tobacco smoking and participation of the overweight in weight control programs. The role of dietary management in the prevention of cardiovascular disease is important. It should be fully understood by the nutritionist providing direct services in agencies, or acting as a consultant to physicians or special heart disease programs. Patients with *simple dietary lipidemia* (see page 207) normally respond to a reduction of their carbohydrate and cholesterol intake. *Familial hyperchylomicronemia* may also be alleviated in the same way; still further improvement in this type of patient may be achieved by substituting fats in the diet with triglycerides of medium chain length that are absorbed directly into the portal circulation. How feasible long-term control by this latter method would be is speculative. When the lipidemia is *carbohydrate ac-*

14*

centuated a reduction in the carbohydrate content of the diet will usually be followed by lowering of the serum triglyceride levels; the effect on cholesterol levels may be less marked. In order to lower cholesterol levels, it may be necessary to reduce the fat and cholesterol in the diet, and substitute saturated fats with unsaturated cholesterol-free fats. Again, there may be practical difficulties in preparing diets which control the lipidemia and yet remain acceptable over a long period of time. *Familial hypercholesterolemia* is usually highly resistant to diet therapy. Nevertheless, the effects of reducing dietary carbohydrates, saturated fats, and foods containing cholesterol should be observed for several months before it is concluded that diet therapy is ineffective. After this, pharmacological agents should be tried. These agents increase the excretion of bile acids and encourage the breakdown of endogenous cholesterol to bile acids.

While there can be no doubt about the efficiency of diet therapy in some cases, it has not been established that the lowering of cholesterol levels has an effect on subsequent cardiovascular morbidity and mortality.

In several studies, patients who survived a coronary heart attack have been placed on diets containing unsaturated vegetable oils. Their subsequent experience of heart disease has been compared with control groups. In general, results have been encouraging but in an experiment in London, it was concluded that the relapse rate from heart attacks was not materially affected by the unsaturated fat content of the diet.[60] The differences in the findings in the various research efforts around the world may be explained by differences in the duration of the experimental period, and the inability to control other risk factors such as smoking and stress.

Other studies have attempted to show the effect of diets containing unsaturated fats on cardiovascular disease in subjects living in institutions and in cities. In a trial on men in the United States, serum cholesterol levels were lowered and there was less sudden death and myocardial infarction in the experimental group but the difference was not statistically significant.[61] When the experience for both heart disease and cerebral infarction were compared however, the experimental group had a significantly lower morbidity and mortality than controls. A similar experiment in New York City among free living males is producing comparable results and it is concluded that the dietary treatment reduces the risk of coronary heart disease.

In the National Diet Heart Study in the United States, it has been found that serum cholesterol levels in free living populations can be lowered by substituting saturated fats with unsaturated vegetable oils.[62]

It is still not known whether a decrease in blood cholesterol levels of the small magnitude that was noted in the above experiments would prevent heart attacks. It should be remembered that the replacement of saturated fats by unsaturated vegetable oils would involve a major revision of shopping, cooking, and eating habits. There would also have to be considerable nutrition education built into the program. It is not generally realized that many foods recommended because they raise the protein content of the diet also raise its fat content. The housewife who prepares the food also needs to be taught the many food sources of cholesterol and some simple but little known facts. For example, she should know that if the oil in margarine is hydrogenated, the cholesterol lowering effect is reduced.

At the present time there seems to be little scientific justification for special nutrition services for the prevention of cardiovascular disease. In view of the uncertainty of the relationship between diet and heart disease, nutrition education and diet counselling should be less dogmatic until more is known of the cause and prevention of this disease. In the meantime possibly the best advice available is to keep physically fit. This implies that the inactive should be persuaded to take more exercise and utilize recreation facilities or local "Jogging Clubs". The overweight should participate in weight control programs.

Rehabilitation and treatment of protein calorie malnutrition

Economic considerations   Medical treatment of disease has been practised for thousands of years but the concept of prevention of disease and promotion of health is a relatively recent phenomenon. This undoubtedly helps to explain why so much emphasis is placed on curative services. Increasing attention has been paid to preventing disease but preventive medicine, public health, and the even newer concept of promotion of health, have not had a fair share of government budgets. With increasing costs of medical care, economy of services is becoming increasingly important as a determinant of the type of care to be provided.

Protein calorie malnutrition provides an excellent example of the high cost of medical treatment and the lower costs of prevention. In examining costs of care, the economic considerations should include all children suffering directly from malnutrition, or indirectly through its synergism with infections. The cost of disease should be related to the costs of all the medical care services. This includes care offered by the government or agency, and the cost of medical care to the parents. This latter not only includes medical fees and transport costs, but also loss of work time. The cost of the child's life must also be taken into consideration; this includes the food consumed by the mother before delivery, and the cost of food, clothing, and shelter in the postnatal period.

Both malnutrition and the synergistic infectious diseases can cause severe handicapping which places an added burden on the society. For example, xeropthalmia as a complication of vitamin A deficiency causes much childhood blindness and places a considerable imposition on the community. Tuberculosis may be complicated by severe physical deformities and loss of function. The effects of inadequate mental development as a result of severe protein calorie malnutrition may be very great in the individual. Whole populations may be comprised of many individuals who have experienced milder forms of malnutrition; this may be one of the reasons why developing countries fail to progress. More studies are required to show the cost of malnutrition; data from such research may help to convince administrators of the soundness of economic investment in the promotion of health.

Where there is a high incidence of malnutrition in the community, the economics of treatment must be examined. It is inevitable that severe cases of malnutrition require the skilled medical and nursing care that can only be obtained in hospitals. However, more cases of protein calorie malnutrition are being diagnosed earlier, and milder cases are being referred to hospitals.

The cost of treatment in hospitals of a severe case of protein calorie malnutrition may be three times the cost of treatment of the mild case. This is because the nutrients and supervision that the mild case requires may be given as an outpatient (see Table 93). The cost of outpatient treatment, and rehabilitation of the child in a special rehabilitation center, may be about one-hundredth of the cost of inpatient care.[63]

Table 93   Comparative costs of services for protein calorie malnutrition

Type of service	Cost per dollar per day
Inpatient treatment—general hospital	4.05
Outpatient treatment—general hospital	1.51
Nutritional Rehabilitation Center	0.89

Source: Beghin, I. D., *Amer. J. Clin. Nutr.* **23**: 1412, 1970.

It is clearly wasteful of resources to rehabilitate a child to health and then return it to home conditions that were responsible for the disease in the first place. The treatment of protein calorie malnutrition has to be supplemented, therefore, by after-care, involving follow-up and education of the parent.

Care and treatment of protein calorie malnutrition   The t...
tein calorie malnutrition is based on the provision of nu...
lacking in the diet, namely good quality protein and ad...
The implementation of this simple regime is far from easy in...
severe cases may have cardiac or gastro-intestinal complicatic...
bolism of patients may be so disturbed that recovery may b...
Even with good hospital care, severe cases have a high mortality, specialized
units report a mortality rate of 15 per cent of admissions.[64] The protein
in the diet is usually provided by dried skimmed milk or, when the economic
situation permits, by casein. Equally good results can be obtained using
either protein source. Gastric upsets that have been associated with the use
of dried skim milk are not due to the milk but to the sugar that is added
to meet the calorie requirement. In protein calorie malnutrition there may
be a deficiency of enzymes which split disaccharides. The subsequent intolerance of the digestive system to sugar may precipitate a terminal and
fatal diarrhea. The calories should be provided by any locally available
vegetable oil such as corn oil, safflower oil, cotton seed oil, or peanut oil.
Despite the digestive disturbances that are a feature of protein calorie
malnutrition, the oil is well tolerated. Much of the success of therapy
depends on the techniques used to administer the milk and oil mixture.
These techniques will be discussed in further detail later.

Infection is an important factor in the ecology and etiology of protein
calorie malnutrition. Children may be admitted to a hospital because of
diarrhea. If this is very severe, the child may be dehydrated and require
intravenous fluid therapy. Diarrhea complicating protein calorie malnutrition may have a dual etiology. The first example is the child who has
been suffering from chronic malnutrition perhaps for weeks, months, or
even longer. Eventually his digestive function is so disturbed that he is
unable to tolerate even plain cereal gruels; diarrhea then supervenes. The
other case is the child who may be suffering from marginal nutrition. In
this type of case, an attack of gastro-enteritis that would not debilitate a
healthy child may precipitate overt malnutrition and severe diarrhea. The
acute onset of this latter type of case causes confusion with the infective ga-
stro enteritis which is so prevalent in infancy in developing countries. The fluid
and electrolyte needs of the child with infective diarrhea may be entirely
different from the child with diarrhea of nutritional origin; therefore a
correct diagnosis is essential. The electrolyte balance in protein calorie malnutrition may be greatly disturbed; these changes must be understood if children
with diarrhea are to be given the correct therapy. The following discussion
is based on the observations and recommendations of Garrow et al. [65]

The malnourished child is actually overhydrated and contains too much water in proportion to his body weight. Even when gastro-enteritis complicates malnutrition, it is rare for the total body water to be decreased below normal body proportions. The cells may be dehydrated but the extracellular fluid more than makes up for this deficiency. In malnutrition, there has been loss of tissue so that the body has an appearance of being dehydrated. However, the situation is very much different from the child with gastro-enteritis for in the latter case there has been no loss of tissue and the extracellular volume is decreased. These differences are of vital clinical importance because the child with gastro-enteritis may die for want of fluid and the malnourished child may die if given fluid.

The malnourished child is potassium depleted (see Figure 125). This is believed to be due to a failure of the kidney to conserve potassium and not to dietary depletion. There may be an almost complete loss of potassium from brain tissue, although blood levels may be normal. The significance of the loss of brain potassium is not understood but it may be responsible for the mental changes that are a feature of severe malnutrition. It is possible that a mechanism exists in healthy persons which maintains potassium in the cells; this may be lost in malnutrition.

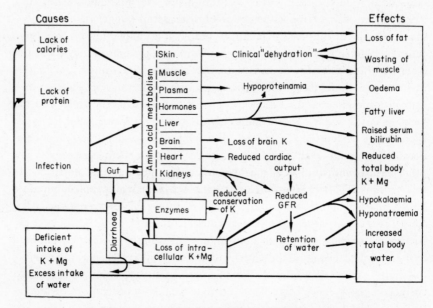

Figure 125   Suggested relations between causes and effects in severe infantile malnutrition (Reproduced from *Electrolyte Balance in Severe Infantile Malnutrition* by J. S. Garrow, R. Smith and E. Ward, 1968, published by Pergamon Press)

The malnourished child is believed to be deficient in magnesium but the exact cause of this phenomenon is not known. Some diets (such as those based on a cassava staple) may be deficient in magnesium; in addition, there may be excessive losses in the urine or in the feces. The function of the cell membranes may be disturbed, consequently the magnesium gradient between the cell and the extracellular fluid may not be maintained. Sodium levels in the blood of the severely malnourished child tends to be subnormal. As the osmotic pressure between the cells and the extracellular fluid depends to a large extent on the sodium, the cells and the extracellular fluids are also hypotonic. Low blood levels of sodium can be caused either by deficits of sodium in the body, or overhydration. As sodium can replace some of the intracellular potassium, deficits of potassium may also be the cause of hyponatremia. In most cases, it is probable that all, or a combination of some, of these factors may be at work.

The prognosis in protein calorie malnutrition can be predicted to some extent from the biochemistry of the blood. The child that is most likely to die has hyponatremia, low blood potassium levels, and raised serum bilirubin levels; the last being indicative of liver damage. The presence of infection with malnutrition carries additional risk because infections by themselves tend to lower serum sodium levels. The malnourished child is therefore in need of potassium but not sodium; the excess of sodium in the body needs to be redistributed to correct the hyponatremia. In theory, the intracellular deficiency of potassium can be corrected by giving potassium chloride, this would then allow the sodium in the cell to leave and re-enter the blood thereby correcting the hyponatremia. In practice, this simple procedure has dangers because of the toxic properties of potassium when given in excess. Intravenous administration of potassium chloride should only be given if blood potassium levels can be determined. Infusions should be limited so that the blood potassium does not exceed 6 mEq per liter. Oral administration of 6–8 mEq of potassium chloride per kg body weight per day in divided doses has been recommended. The retention of potassium may be facilitated by giving magnesium. When the electrolyte balance is restored, the water retention in the body should be relieved. It has been recommended that the child be deprived of food and water but the effectiveness and safety of this recommendation has not yet been established.

Administration of sodium is contra-indicated since the child already has an excess of this mineral that it cannot excrete adequately. Despite the excess of total body water, diarrhea may reduce the plasma volume to dangerous levels so that intravenous therapy may be indicated to restore the plasma volume.

The differentiation of the child with gastro-enteritis from the malnourished child with dehydration is critical for the former may require fluids and sodium; the latter may be seriously harmed if given sodium and it may, or may not, have needs for fluids. In both types of cases there may be weight loss, pallor, a greyish discoloration of the skin, loss of tissue turgor, lethargy, and subnormal temperature. In true dehydration however, the mucous membranes are dry and in young infants the anterior fontanelle may be depressed. The pulse is usually weak and rapid in dehydration.

The malnourished child with diarrhea requires much less fluid than that usually given to dehydrated infants with gastro-enteritis. The pulse should be used as a therapeutic guide and infusion should stop when the pulse slows. Half-strength Darrows solution with 2.5 per cent dextrose produces good results; 4 per cent sodium bicarbonate may be added for infants with acidosis. In view of the dangers of giving sodium to a "sodium loaded" child, the presence of sodium chloride in the urine would be a definite contra-indication for therapy with saline solutions. The sodium chloride may be detected by the silver nitrate test.

A review of the types of therapy used in protein calorie malnutrition shows that there is a diversity of opinion on the use of intravenous therapy.[66] It has been suggested that the varying success of different therapeutic regimes may be explained by geographic variation in the disease.

Protein calorie malnutrition may be further complicated by liver failure, cardiac failure, anemia, and infections. Liver failure may not be discernable clinically in its early stages, but biochemically it is indicated by a rise in serum bilirubin levels. Autopsies on cases dying from liver failure have revealed potassium deficits. It has been suggested that an intake of 1 gram potassium chloride per kg body weight per day should be achieved when there is evidence of liver failure. Infections should be treated with antibiotics, and anemia by ferrous sulfate and folic acid. It should be remembered that the anemia of kwashiorkor may not appear until the child has been under treatment for some time.[67] Therefore, hemoglobin levels should be measured regularly during treatment. Disturbances in cardiac function have been attributed to magnesium deficiency which is aggravated by high intakes of protein, calcium, phosphorus, and possibly potassium. Magnesium salts may be given orally as magnesium hydroxide. The patient must be adequately hydrated however, as dangerously high levels can accumulate in the dehydrated state. In severe cases where oral therapy may be inadequate, it should be given intramuscularly. Magnesium should not be given intravenously, since it can cause dangerous hypotension.

A 50 per cent solution of $MgSO_4 . 7H_2O$ (Epsom salts) is recommended. One ml contains 49 mg or 4 mEq of magnesium; 0.5 ml is usually considered adequate for infants weighing between 4 and 7 kg. Heavier children may be given 1 ml.

The care and skilled nursing that protein calorie malnutrition demands has led to the development of specialized units termed *malwards*. These are now being incorporated into hospitals in areas where protein calorie malnutrition is prevalent. They represent an important advance in providing specialized care that demands neither highly trained manpower, nor expensive equipment. A *malward* is useful also in linking up treatment, after care, and preventive services.

The function and operation of malwards   A child with severe malnutrition requires varying types of care and treatment, according to its clinical state and nutritional needs. These needs vary during the acute illness, recovery, and rehabilitation. Treatment in *malwards* can be considered in four phases. The first is *rehydration* (where this is necessary), the second is *intensive care*, the third *high protein-high calorie feeding* and the last, *rehabilitation and follow-up*.[68]

Rehydration. Severe cases of malnutrition may be complicated by diarrhea and many infants and children are admitted to "gastro-intestinal wards". The principles of care and management in this phase have already been discussed.

Intensive care and milk formula feeding. In this phase, the nutritional needs are met, and the electrolyte balance is restored by appropriate potassium and magnesium therapy. The basis of the immediate therapy is the provision of a dried skim milk and vegetable oil mixture that provides ample protein of good quality and source of calories. Table 94 shows the composition of a typical milk-oil mixture; 125 ml of this formula provides approximately four grams of protein and 115 calories. This basic formula may be diluted to provide levels of three, two or one gram of protein per kg of body weight per day. Since the mineral intake will be reduced by dilution, the original concentration of magnesium and potassium salts should be restored. Many of the infants are fretful and irritable; attempts to bottle feed or spoon feed a struggling child may add further stress and lead to a dangerous state of exhaustion. Diarrhea also contra-indicates feeding large quantities of food at one time. For these reasons the child should be mildly sedated, and fed through an intragastric tube. It has been found that giving the milk-oil mixture as a "drip" is a convenient way to administer the therapy continuously and to control the amount given. When diarrhea is very severe the milk-oil mixture may be diluted. The amount and concentration of the mixture is increased or decreased as necessary according to the number of stools passed daily. This phase of the care requires constant attention and careful recording of the food intake. Usually after 36 to 48 hours the tube can be removed and the mixture fed by bottle or cup. The child should by this time be on full strength milk-oil mixtures and consuming approximately 4 grams protein per kg body weight per day.

Table 94   Composition of basic milk and oil mixture

Item	Quantity (g)	Protein Content (g)	Calorie Content
Dried Skim Milk	93.0	31.8	321
Vegetable Oil	68.0	0	612
Magnesium hydroxide	1.2	0	0
Potassium chloride	4.0	0	0
	166.2	31.8	933

Add water to 1000 grams.

If edema is being lost there may be some loss of weight at this time. When a steady weight gain has been achieved, the child may be given a full strength cows milk formula preparatory to the next phase of therapy.

High protein, high calorie diet. The milk diet is replaced by one prepared from local foods providing a high concentration of protein and calories.

The first solid foods should be introduced at the time of day when full attention can be given to tempting the child to eat. Menus involving a wide variety of foods should be available so the child may be offered a choice. A careful record should be kept of food consumed, and food left over or wasted, to enable the daily protein and calorie intake to be estimated.

Meals consisting of the milk formula should be replaced with solid foods; if there is intolerance to solids then the milk mixtures should be re-introduced. The food should be offered *ad libitum*; a decline in the appetite should be expected as therapy progresses. When it can be seen that the child is making satisfactory progress, low cost foods which may form the bulk of the diet in the home situation are introduced into the diet.

Low cost diet. The menu offered in this phase of treatment is based on inexpensive protein foods, many dishes include legumes. Mothers tend to believe that beans and peas are unsuited for child feeding consequently, a certain amount of practical nutrition education is needed. By getting the mother to feed the child, there is a better change of her being convinced of the acceptability of the food. She is given instruction on homecraft, infant care, and the preparation of low cost, nutritious foods. This instruction may be given by specially trained aides who assist the hospital dietitian. Throughout the entire hospitalization of the patient, progress should be evaluated by increase in body weight. This should be measured daily in the early stages of the disease. Skinfold thickness and other anthropometric measurements should be recorded regularly and hemoglobin levels should be determined weekly. If biochemical tests can be made, serum transferrin and serum protein levels provide useful measures of progress.

Follow-up. When the child is discharged, he should be returned to home conditions that are capable of maintaining adequate health and nutrition. The follow-up procedure should not be looked on solely as a means of surveillance since it can play a very positive role in health promotion. For example, it should assist parents to obtain help, relief, or financial support needed to keep the whole family in good health. Since conditions which debilitate one member of the family may be debilitating others too, it should be used as an opportunity to monitor the health of siblings and other relatives. An appraisal of the home situation may help to identify poor environmental conditions responsible for perpetuating bouts of diarrhea, or parasitic infestations.

The follow-up should be used also to educate professionals and it should involve physicians (or medical students) and nurses (or student nurses). The experience should help them to learn better ways to prevent malnutrition by an understanding of the ecology and etiology of the disease. Finally, the follow-up should be used to encourage coordination between the agencies that provide medical, health, education, welfare and food services for the community. This will entail the introduction of an administrative procedure that will notify staff of the participating units who may be called on to help the child and the family.

On discharge from the hospital, a referral letter or report should be made to the *rural health unit* (or center) serving the family (see Figure 126). Further contacts may be made with the local school teacher and the local welfare service which may be able to assist indigent or broken families. It may be necessary to call on local voluntary agencies for help in providing food or diet supplements. If an *applied nutrition program* or comprehensive care project is situated near the child's home, then they may also be called on to provide material help, advice, or education. It should not be overlooked that poverty and large families may be the principle cause of family breakdown so *family planning services* may be important for preventing malnutrition.

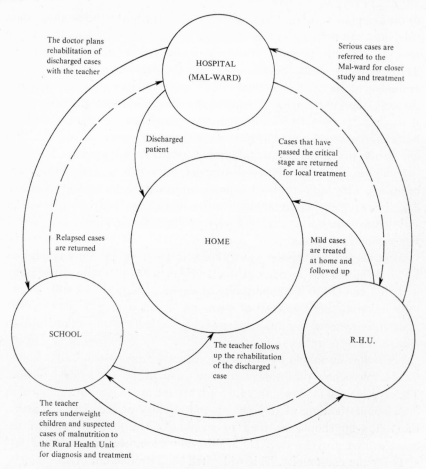

The doctor plans
rehabilitation of
discharged cases
with the teacher

HOSPITAL
(MAL-WARD)

Serious cases are
referred to the
Mal-ward for closer
study and treatment

Discharged
patient

Cases that have
passed the critical
stage are returned
for local treatment

Relapsed cases
are returned

HOME

Mild cases
are treated
at home and
followed up

SCHOOL

R.H.U.

The teacher follows
up the rehabilitation
of the discharged
case

The teacher
refers underweight
children and suspected
cases of malnutrition to
the Rural Health Unit
for diagnosis and treatment

Figure 126   The Referral System (Figure adapted from original by Dr. F. Solon Cebu, Philippines

In many developing countries, resources are limited. Hospitals may be inadequate in number, or they may be unequally distributed throughout the population. In such circumstances the main preventive and curative services have to be based in the *dispensary* or the *rural health center*. The development of outpatient care of malnourished infants now enables malnourished children to receive nutritional rehabilitation and so relieve the load on overburdened hospitals.

Nutrition rehabilitation centers   There are two main types of *nutritional rehabilitation center*. The first treats children as outpatients, and the second accepts the child and the mother as residents.

The day nutrition rehabilitation center. The organization of a center is similar to that of a *creche* or *day care center.* The children are referred from an outpatient clinic or dispensary to the center and they spend most of the day there. In a typical center, the children are given a dried skim milk-oil mixture. If the child is fretful it may be sedated and fed by intra-gastric tube and drop. At the and of the day the mother takes the child home for the night and brings him back the following day. At first the mother naturally experiences some anxiety for the welfare of her child and she is allowed to remain with the child. Usually she becomes reassured quite quickly and she helps to prepare the food and meals for other con-valescent children. In this way she learns how to make low cost weaning foods from local protein sources. She is also given instruction in infant care, correct infant feeding practices, and homecraft. This type of center

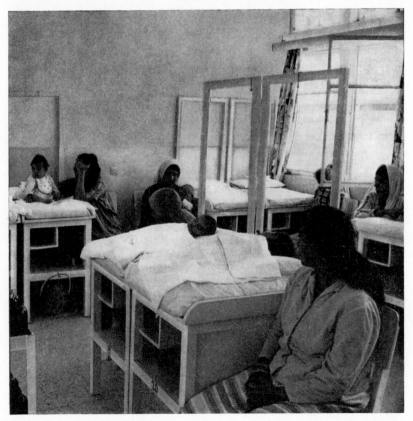

Plate 33   A day rehabilitation center in Jordan. Mothers stay with the child during rehabilitation (WHO photograph)

does not require highly specialized personnel, provided the basic staff are well trained in their duties. In some areas where marasmus is the main problem, the infants are in a younger age group and may be suffering from diarrhea and disturbances in electrolyte balance. Because of this the center should be provided with medical supervision.

The residential rehabilitation center. This type of center is usually found in urban areas. It requires highly trained staff and it serves as a convalescent center. Although the hospital *malward* may be taking over the role of the *residential rehabilitation center*, the latter are particularly useful for the care of infants and children who live some distance away from the hospital.

The emphasis is on the provision of high protein, high calorie foods of local origin. The mother is involved also in the care of the child, the running of the center, and in informal education. This last item includes infant feeding, better weaning practices, the preparation of weaning foods, and nutritious food for the toddler.

There are problems inherent in the management of protein calorie malnutrition that will continue to limit the use of *rehabilitation centers*. The time required for rehabilitation may be in the region of four to six weeks. The education of the mother also takes some time and there is a tendency for the mother to abscond before the infant has fully recovered. The effectiveness of *rehabilitation centers* in scattered rural populations is also doubtful. It has been suggested that *day rehabilitation centers* should be used only in populations of 2000 or more.[63] There is a risk of infection being passed from child to child but with proper supervision this hazard can be minimized.

The *nutritional rehabilitation center* should be not considered as an integral part of a health center. In many situations it may be convenient to include a rehabilitation unit in a health center but this should not mean that *nutritional rehabilitation centers* can not operate independently. The services should meet the need; an urban concentration with a high prevalence of malnutrition may require many more rehabilitation centers than health centers.[69] Generally the *day care center* is preferable to the *residential center* because benefits are high while costs are low. It has been recommended that the *day care center* should be equipped and staffed to treat 30 to 35 children suffering from uncomplicated malnutrition. Medical supervision should be available. The effectiveness of *rehabilitation centers* would be increased if care is taken in the selection of cases. Surveillance at outpatient clinics is not adequate. Screening of children by weight, through services for the preschool child and through home visits, should bring to light other cases that have not become sick enough to warrant a visit to the outpatient department of a hospital. Cases of this degree of severity may be more quickly restored to health at less expense. Selection of cases should also pay attention to the family and early identification of the family at risk. In Nigeria a number of characteristics of at-risk families have been defined, including family size, marital state, mortality of siblings, birthweight, and weight gain in the first six months of life. Underweight is more common in children with a birth order above seven, in infants with a birth weight below the tenth percentile. Underweight is also associated with a weight gain of less than one pound in the first three months and less than one-half pound per month in subsequent months.

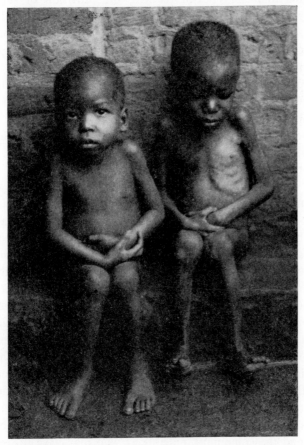

Plate 34   Identifying the marginally nourished. The wasting of the chest and upper arms of the child on the right is obvious. The child on the left is also suffering from protein calorie malnutrition but the signs are less apparent. Children like this may be screened out by routine weighing at clinics (Photograph by Dr. F. J. Brennett).

Families that were characterized by broken marriage or more than four deaths were also likely to have malnourished children.[70]

This type of information can be collected by various categories of public health personnel during clinic or home visits. The significance of the data should be communicated to those responsible for advising mothers on infant feeding practices.

As in the case of *malwards*, a good follow-up service is essential and the rehabilitation unit should be part of overall services which protect and promote the health of the infant and child (see Figure 126). The rehabilitation unit is one part of an overall program that includes the expansion of maternal and child health services, the provision of supplementary foods, the development of new protein sources, education of the public in nutrition, and the raising of economic standards. Rehabilitation units also help to develop collaboration between the various departments, and ministries, whose activities contribute to the provision of more and better food, better nutrition, and better social and economic standards of living.

Before closing this discussion on specialized services for infants, children, and youth, it may be useful to summarize the objectives of a nutrition clinic. These are based on a review of the services offered in many parts of the world.

Nutrition clinics   Clinics should provide services which keep surveillance over the nutritional status of the infant, child, and youth population. They should promote better nutrition, prevent malnutrition, and they should be actively involved in the management of malnutrition.[71] The service should assist in bringing total care to the young, and should include social as well as health care. The clinic should act as a bridge between the hospital *milieu* and the community. It should assist in the translation of therapeutic regimes into feasible dietary practices that will continue to restore and maintain health in the malnourished. Nutrition clinics should provide a medium for bringing the disciplines together. For example, the child who is failing to thrive may be suffering because of an emotional problem in the mother. The nutritional problem in this case should bring together the psychiatrist in community mental health, the nutritionist, and the pediatrician. The clinic should make nutrition counselling available to patients and their families. It should help to bridge the gap between the clinician and the community nutritionist who may have to deal with the same problems in two entirely different environments. The clinic should serve as a training ground for physicians, nurses, and dietitians in the subspeciality of pediatric nutrition. It should offer training in the clinical aspects of childhood nutrition to professional and sub-professionals in the field of nutrition, social work, extension, and anthropology. The nutrition clinic should serve as a center for the evaluation of growth, emotional maturation, and intellectual function. It should provide biochemical, biophysical, and biostatistical data which may be used to establish ranges of normality. It should serve as a center for the evaluation of services and their effect on growth and nutritional status.

Special community services and projects

Specific problems within the community may determine the type of services required. Some problems may be so serious that special services have to be developed to introduce some measure of control. If one particular disease does not demand special attention, priorities may have to be established by appraising mortality data or morbidity patterns of cases admitted to hospitals or clinics. In a survey of child inpatients in a hospital in Sierra Leone, the principal causes of death give some guidance on priorities for programs and services[72] (see Table 95).

Table 95 Principal causes of death in a Sierra Leone Hospital

Disease	Percentage of total deaths
Pneumonia	24
Diarrhea	17
Malaria	15
Malnutrition	11
Tetanus	10
Severe anemia	9
Measles and sequelae	8
Native medicine intoxication	5
Encephalitis	3
Whooping cough	2
Tuberculosis	2

Source: Wilkinson, J. L. *Trans. Roy. Soc. Trop. Med. and Hyg.* **63**: 263, 1969.

Local patterns of morbidity may emphasize certain diseases whose importance may be lost in the overall national data. In the hospital in Sierra Leone, infections of one sort or another, accounted for 49 per cent of all deaths. In view of the synergism between infection and malnutrition, it may be appreciated that combined disease control and efforts to promote

15*

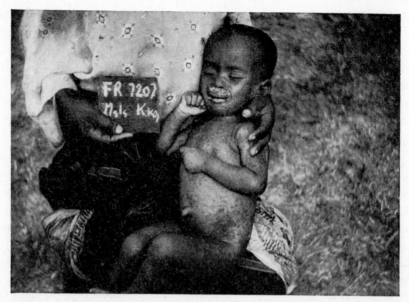

Plate 35   Synergism between infection and malnutrition. This Nigerian child developed
kwashiorkor after an attack of measles. The skin is affected all over the body, unlike
kwashiorkor which has not been preceded by measles. The seriousness of the illness
indicates the need for combined disease control and improved nutrition (Photograph
by Dr. David Morley)

better nutrition may have a considerable impact on mortality experience
in that geographical area.

   Community nutrition problems have motivated the development of a
multidisciplinary approach known as *applied nutrition programs*. Usually
these have the specific objective of reducing the incidence of protein calorie
malnutrition in a target community.

Applied nutrition programs   These have been sponsored by the specialized
agencies of the United Nations such as the World Health Organization,
the United Nations Children Fund, and the Food and Agriculture Organization. The Philippines Bayambang Project is typical of one such project.[73]
Based on a *Normal School* (Teacher Training College), the community
and the children attending the "laboratory" school were involved in food
production, the preparation and provision of school snacks, improved
methods of agriculture and horticulture, and education including budgeting,
meal planning, and home food production.

   These projects are difficult to administer because three international
agencies may be involved, in addition to national and provincial government

agencies. The effectiveness of *applied nutrition programs* is also difficult to evaluate. This special problem will be discussed in detail later in this chapter.

Applied nutrition programs originated from various activities initiated by the United Nations Special Agencies, World Health Organization, the Food and Agriculture Organization, and the United Nations Childrens Fund. All of these agencies were becoming increasingly involved in cooperative action against protein calorie malnutrition some 15 years ago. Their programs at first had two major emphases, strengthening national nutrition services and group feeding.

Their efforts were inadequate and in 1957 UNICEF extended the scope of its aid to include assistance to nutrition surveys, training, education,

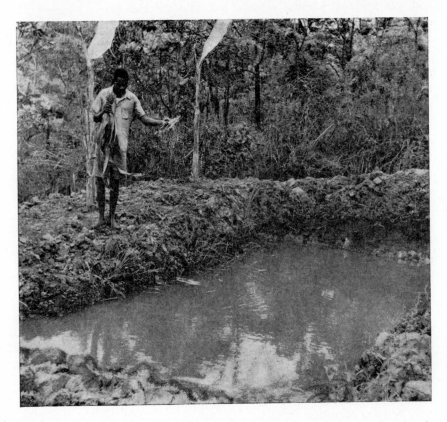

Plate 36   Applied nutrition. Domestic fish production in the Maposeni project in Songea District, Tanzania. A pond of this size stocked with *Tilapia*, a member of the carp family, can provide a family with a useful source of good quality protein. The fish are being fed banana leaves taken from plants growing on the banks of the pond (FAO photograph)

horticulture, fish and poultry production, and supplementary feeding. These programs became known as *applied nutrition programs*. By 1966, sixty programs had been started in thirty-five countries.

Assistance towards the establishment of an *applied nutrition program* is initiated by a government request to the specialized agencies of the United Nations. *A plan of operations* is drafted and approved by WHO, FAO and UNICEF who usually supply personnel, supplies, and equipment. *Applied nutrition programs* may not necessarily involve international assistance. Programs with virtually the same function have been developed in some countries on national resources alone. The Maposeni project, described in the introduction to this book was a forerunner of *applied nutrition programs* and was operated without external aid. Many similar projects have been started in other countries; some of them have been developed with bilateral aid.

Often, progress has been hindered by lack of coordination of government activities, by lack of trained staff, and lack of nutritionally important foods in the community at prices acceptable to the family budget. In *applied nutrition programs* many attempts have been made to encourage food production. However, the local staple proved to be in short supply in some programs and could not be produced in sufficient quantities to meet the needs. In other programs a glut of food was produced which could not be absorbed by the community. The seasonal availability of some foods in the production program raised problems.

The projects have a secondary intention of coordinating government, private, and public bodies whose function is to help the population to learn to produce food and consume a better diet. The programs are also intended to study, test, and popularize educational methods and techniques and they also serve as a training facility. The organization of the programs has proved to be formidable since there has to be a central integrating and co-ordinating body. In some instances this is the *National Coordinating Committee on Food and Nutrition*. There has to be also a de-centralized body in the region where the program is executed and finally an executive body is needed at the project site. Each of these administrative bodies are multi-disciplinary and the complexity of the organization may be judged from Figures 127 and 128 which show the organization of the Philippines Bayambang Applied Nutrition Project.

Experience with *applied nutrition programs* has shown that the equilibrium between agriculture, health, and education is soon lost and one of the authorities assumes more responsibility than others. Many of the programs develop according to the particular interests of international experts. This

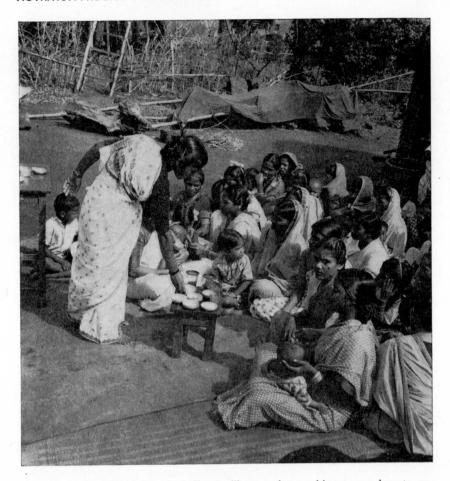

Plate 37   Applied nutrition in India. A village worker teaching women how to prepare nutritious meals in Orissa, India. (FAO photograph by Jack Ling)

is understandable since many of the projects are geographically isolated and there is little opportunity for an exchange of knowledge between staff of the various programs. Recruitment of experts for international work is far from easy. In addition, strangers may not be acceptable in some isolated countries, and there may be cultural barriers to surmount.

The future of *applied nutrition programs* is uncertain; the large scale operation may become more of a rarity but there is evidence that some of them are serving a useful purpose. In the Philippines there has been a remarkable expansion of activities. The original project in Bayambang was succeeded by other projects that have been established in other provinces

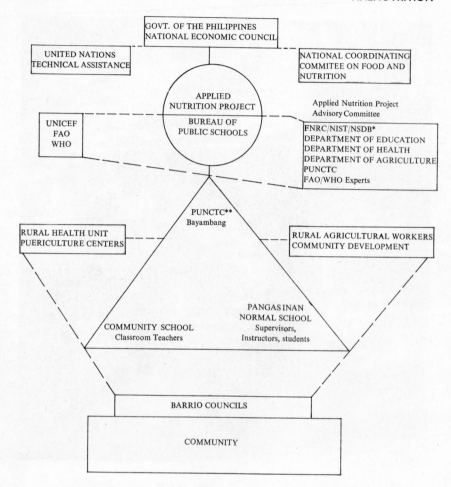

Figure 127   Organizational chart of the Philippines Applied Nutrition Program

and islands. There are now over 225 schools involved in applied nutrition projects as part of the Philippines *applied nutrition program.* Training of staff and community leaders and the introduction of applied nutrition courses in five regional teacher training colleges has been a major activity. A total of 5400 government officials and 4200 members of the community had been trained between July 1964 and February 1969. This was a sure objective sign of government and community involvement in the program.

ACTION CHANNEL FOR HEALTH DEPARTMENT PERSONNEL
PHILIPPINES APPLIED NUTRITION PROGRAM

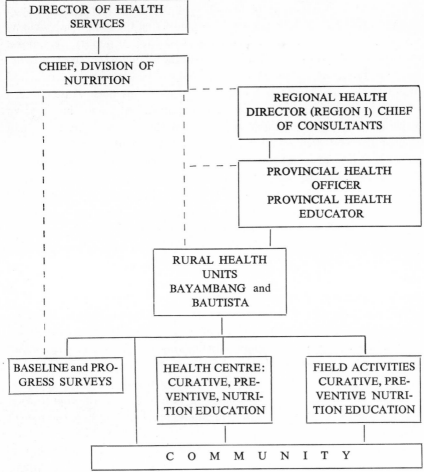

Figure 128   Organizational chart

National and international food programs A full discussion of food programs is not possible in this text. Since nutritionists are frequently involved in the execution of these programs at the local level some of the concepts of these programs will be reviewed in brief.

While population planning programs continue to try to bring the increase in the world population under control, considerable efforts must be expended to increase the world food supply to meet the needs of the growing population.

The Food and Agriculture Organization has developed an integrated program to close the gap between population growth and food production; it is entitled *The Indicative World Plan for Agricultural Development.*[74] The plan has two stages; in the first, priority is given to increasing the yield per unit area. This is to be achieved by intensifying the use of high yielding varieties of cereals. At the same time the production of poultry, eggs, pork, milk, beef, veal, and other meat is urged. In the second stage, cereal production is to be expanded less rapidly, and land will be used for the production of other crops and livestock. Some of these proposals must cause concern when their practical implications are examined. Although increases in yields may be highly desirable they often result in a decrease in protein content per unit area of production. Quantity should not be considered alone. It is also essential to insure that the quality of the protein is high. Communities may not adopt high yielding varieties of cereals just because they are made available (see page 152). The use of animal products, as protein concentrates, is an excellent arrangement provided the animals are not being fed on products which humans could utilize, or being raised on land that could be used for growing food for direct human consumption. The conversion of plant protein into animal protein is inefficient (see page 153), which raises doubts as to the wisdom of advising increases in production of beef, veal, and other meat.

The plan assumes that there is, or will be, communications, markets, and distributing systems and a population anxious and willing to consume the produce. Although the hungry and starving are unlikely to refuse food, it must not be forgotten that humans have minds and opinions of their own. There is no guarantee that this theoretically correct advice will be accepted on a global scale and it may be naive to believe that it will change food intake patterns. The problems of bringing about change in food habits will be discussed in the next chapter.

National and international programs are exploring the exploitation of novel sources of protein. It is apparent that no single source of protein is likely to satisfy the impending need. Leaf protein concentrates, microbial protein, or the production of protein from fossil fuels, have not only economic and technological problems, but they will also have to face the problem of acceptability to humans. It has been suggested that more attention should be paid to exploiting and developing existing sources of protein that are known to be acceptable.[75] Amaranth and sweet potato leaves are examples of many green leaves that give high yields of protein. Unfortunately other varieties of vegetables such as tomato tend to be encouraged because they are more familiar to "Experts" from temperate regions of the world who are employed as advisors to governments in tropical areas.

The use of protein materials for the supplementary feeding of children is the subject of much research. Because of the potential dangers of experiments involving the feeding of malnourished infants, much of the research is guided and coordinated by the *Protein Advisory Group*. It is composed of representatives of WHO, FAO, UNICEF, and UNESCO. The group is currently concerned with the nature and magnitude of the *protein gap*. This is the deficiency between the supply and demand for protein, by the world population. Other subjects under discussion include, amino acid fortification, toxic substances in new protein foods, marketing of protein supplements, and feeding the preschool child. Guidelines are published for the methodology of pre-clinical and clinical testing of materials.

Food materials that are constantly under review include *single cell proteins* and supplementary food prepared from oil, seeds, and nuts and "milk-like" products.[76] The features of the last named have already been discussed (see page 130). *Single cell protein (SCP)* is not a new concept in human feeding. Algae from Lake Chad has been used as a source of food in Africa for centuries. SCP may originate from bacteria protozoa, yeasts, fungi, or algae. When these are grown on a suitable medium there is a yield of cells containing 35–75 per cent of protein, suitable as a source of food. Although the lysine content of SCP is satisfactory, the protein is deficient in the sulfur amino acids. Bacteria and yeasts appear to offer the best potential source of SCP.

Single cell protein can be grown on inexpensive substrates such as waste carbohydrate material, or hydrocarbons, including gas oil and methane. They may require only the addition of nitrogen, phosphorus, some minerals, water, and air. The cells grow rapidly and yields can be impressive; however, heat is produced which means the medium requires cooling. Because of this and a variety of other technical, economic, and social considerations, only a small quantity of SCP is being produced at the present time. A wide variety of protein foods have been prepared from oil seed residues (see Table 96). Because of amino imbalances in the proteins, oils seed residues are usually mixed with legumes, cereals, or animal proteins. Previous comments made on the side effects of fortification of cereals with amino acids, are also pertinent to supplementary foods (see page 487). Excesses of a single amino acid are unlikely when the supplement consists of food materials. However, the stimulation of growth by the supplement may lead to secondary nutrient deficiencies. Of more importance, in practice, is the assurance that the diet provides enough calories. If there is a calorie deficiency the protein in the supplement will be used as a source of energy rather than for catabolism. There are many reports of supplementary

Table 96 Protein food mixtures

Product	Country	Composition	Protein content %	NDpCal %
Incaparina	Guatemala	Maize, cotton seed flour, vit. A, lysine CaCO$_3$	27.5	7.4
Pronutro	South Africa	Maize, skim milk, peanut, soya, fish protein concentrate, yeast, wheat germ, vit. A, thiamine, riboflavin, niacin, sugar, iodized salt	22.0	
Saridele	Indonesia	Dry soya, sugar, CaCO$_3$, thiamine, folate, ascorbic acid	26–30	
Arlac	Nigeria	Peanut flour, skim milk, salts, thiamine, riboflavin, folate, vit. D	42.0	
Indian Multi-purpose Food	India	Peanut flour, chickpea flour, CaCO$_3$, vit. A, thiamine, riboflavin	40.0	
C. S. M.	USA	Maize, soya flour, skim milk, CaCO$_3$, vitamins	20.0	10.8
Laubina	Lebanon	Wheat, chickpea, sesame, skim milk, minerals, vit. A and D, thiamine, riboflavin, niacin	16.0	7.8
Fish flour	Chile	Fish flour, butter, lactose, sucrose, cornstarch, vitamins, minerals		7.0

Source: PAG Bulletin No. 7, *Amer. J. Clin. Nutr.* **17**: 143, 1965, and *Proc. Seventh Int'I Congr. Nutr.*, **4**: 152, 1967.

feeding programs being ineffective and it has been suggested that this has been caused by an overall dietary calorie deficiency.[77]

Finally, there must be a recognition of the presence of large numbers of children in developing countries who have an intolerance to lactose. Whether this is a genetic defect, the result of loss of the enzyme after weaning, or to intestinal disease is immaterial.[78,79] The intolerance may mean that well-intentioned supplementation with foods containing milk, may cause a deterioration in health.

Evaluation of nutrition programs and services

Evaluation is necessary for insuring that plans and action are effective and achieving the intended goals. All nutrition programs and services should have, as a general objective, the accomplishment of higher levels of operational efficiency. In turn, the increased efficiency should help to attain better standards of health and nutritional status.

Ideally, the initial plan for a program, or project, should include a methodology for evaluation and periodic reassessment of progress. Unfortunately, many programs and services have been initiated without any real thought being given to evaluation. The problems of assessing the effectiveness of ongoing services will be discussed first. Later, attention will be directed towards the evaluation of new nutrition programs.

Evaluating ongoing health and nutrition programs

Ideally, a study should be established in which achievements of objectives are compared in experimental and control groups of populations. Care must be taken in selecting objectives and measuring progress because they may be subject to influences outside the scope of the service that is being evaluated. A general improvement in health is, liable, for example to be influenced by an amelioration in socio-economic and environmental conditions. Better growth might be as much due to a decrease in infectious disease as improved nutrition. Because of the difficulty in differentiating the respective influences, intermediate goals are frequently defined. One such goal could be the wider use of nutritional knowledge.

Having decided on objectives to be evaluated, the methodology of testing for achievement, utilizing an experimental and control group, is rarely feasible in life. In most situations there are too many variable factors whose influence cannot be assessed. It is, difficult, for example to find two groups that are comparable and accessible yet insulated one from the other, so there are no inter-group influences. Selection of two neighboring populations may introduce bias from differences in socio-economic levels. Selection of a sample within a neighborhood may cause problems because one sample may resent being denied services offered to the other.

Even when testing for intermediate objectives it may be impossible to determine whether achievements are attributable to the activity of nutritionists, nurses, or health educators. The natural desire to be as "scientific" as possible in evaluating progress should not induce the evaluator to try to assess the representative contributions of each professional worker, or to compare the effects of direct counselling or indirect service. The task may be impossible and it may hide the important fact that the public is acquiring information on nutrition.

In many health agencies, the improvement of nutrition is bound up in the activities of various bureaus and divisions and it involves several disciplines. In New York State Department of Health where such problems existed, evaluation of an ongoing program was carried out in three phases.[80] The first phase included an evaluation of existing data, the second was designed to define a methodology for further evaluation. The third phase was to outline needed changes, or innovations, in the existing program. The initial step in the first phase was to categorize the target population. The first category consisted of everyone in the population who would be the target of services designed to reduce morbidity and mortality from nutritional disease. The second category included the vulnerable groups for whom specific activities were planned. These included the infant, child, adolescent, and the pregnant mother who might be in good health but who has to be maintained in that state. The other category was for the sick, including those with chronic disease, obesity, and handicapping conditions.

The categorizing proved to be of value because deficiencies in the existing reporting procedure were revealed immediately. Reports devoted to an account of time spent on general activities in the various divisions and bureaus, were replaced by new ones that included better data related more to the target groups. Whereas formerly, a nursing home was reported from the point of view of an institution, under the new system it was reported as a service for the chronically ill; this placed a better perspective on the goal. Reporting on categories has an additional advantage in that it is likely to induce inter-disciplinary action.

The next phase of the evaluation involved the review of each category, and a justification of each aspect of the program. This required an enumeration of existing activities, evidence of effectiveness, and suggestions for improvement. This method of approach may not appear to be entirely objective, but changes can be introduced for more legitimate reasons than they can when there has been no evaluation.

One of the results of the evaluation of the services offered by the New York State Health Department was the recognition of high maternal mortality in a rural area in New York State. Lowering of this rate was assigned to a team of professionals. These included nutritionists who gave direct counselling to mothers in their homes or in small groups, and who taught nutrition to nurses. Although the contribution of the nutritionist could not be evaluated, this direct, and indirect approach, was very successful. Other benefits started to accrue. For example, the importance of nutrition education became more widely recognized and was introduced into inservice training programs. The level of understanding of nutrition by the public and staff serves as an additional tool for evaluating the effectiveness of the teaching.

While the impact of this limited type of evaluation may not be great, the adoption of a mundane assessment of this kind may lead the way to more effective methodologies.

Evaluating new nutrition programs and services

In many situations a community is served by health services. These, may include the provision of infant and maternal care, the provision of social and welfare services, and voluntary food aid programs. From time to time it is important to assess whether they are effective and still needed.

In 1950, the Philippine government, with assistance from WHO and UNICEF, sponsored a Rural Health Demonstration and Training Center. This was to serve as a practical training station for health staff, and students training in medicine, nursing, and health-related fields.[81] It was intended also, to test and demonstrate procedures for improving health with special emphasis on the mother and child. Novaliches, a District in Quezon City, was selected as the project site. Over a period of ten years, several public health services were introduced including intensive maternal and child health services and domiciliary care that provided a 24-hour midwifery and home delivery service. In addition, there was a school health education program, improved environmental sanitation and communicable disease control. Social welfare was also made available to the population and there was access to good laboratory services for examination of tissue fluids, the detection of parasites, and evaluation of anemia. Health and nutrition education of the public was introduced also into the project.

Before the project was initiated in 1950, baseline data had been gathered in a house to house survey. It was proposed to resurvey the area in 1960 to measure the impact of the project. The evaluation was supplemented by reports from the Training Center and other available related agencies. In order to assess progress, certain health indices had been established in 1950; these were reexamined in 1960 to facilitate comparisons of health over the decennium. The indices included mortality and morbidity rates and the environmental sanitation practices of the population. This latter included the percentage of families with adequate toilet facilities, refuse disposal, and an adequate, safe water supply. The improvement in maternal and child health practices was evaluated by the change in the percentage

of expectant mothers with proper prenatal, natal, and postnatal supervision, and improvements in the care and nutritional status of infants and
preschool children. Changes in the utilization of health resources, improvements in birth registration and improvements in dental health were also
measured.

It was important to establish that the population surveyed in 1950 was
the same as that being resurveyed in 1960 since new immigrants would
invalidate the results. The original survey forms had been incorporated
into family folders and these were traced to check the 1960 population.
Approximately 93 per cent of the original forms and population were
recovered and the resurvey was able to continue. A random sample was
selected and tested to see that it had the same characteristics as the original
population with respect to age, sex, and geographical distribution. Statistical tests confirmed that there were no significant differences in the samples
of the two populations.

A random sample of families was selected and surveyed using the same
schedule, form, and methodology used in 1950. Additional questions were
introduced into the interview to define individuals in the community who
might be classed as *acceptors* or *rejectors* of modern health innovations.
By comparisons with similar persons identified prior to the project, it was
hoped that reasons for an increase in use of health services might come
to light. Special studies included a parasite survey, a dental, clinical, and
anthropometric evaluation, and hemoglobin measurement. Studies were
also made of abnormalities of pregnancy and completeness of birth registration. The results of the two surveys were then compared.

Between 1950 and 1960 there was a decline in general mortality, infant
mortality, and morbidity rates. There was a general decline in the ten leading
causes of death, excepting pneumonia, the leading cause of death in the
Philippines. In 1950 infantile beriberi was the principle cause of death
in childhood. In 1960 this disease no longer appeared as a cause of death;
the change was attributed to better prenatal, natal, and child health supervision. However, it is possible that the diagnosis of death may have improved.
Tuberculosis had decreased, a trend that may have been due to better
chemotherapy, an improved understanding of disease control by the popu-
lace, and improved sanitation. It was noticed that chronic diseases such as
cardiovascular disease and cancer were making an increased contribution
to mortality. This could indicate that the population was living longer,
because of better medical and health care.

There was a significant increase in the improvement of environmental
practices of the people, for example, garbage disposal was better and toilets

had increased in number. In spite of these improvements, gastro-intestinal disease had not declined to any great extent over the ten-year period; this failure may have been due to the lack of a safe municipal water supply.

The improvement in maternal care practices was quite marked; 76.9 per cent of expectant mothers sought prenatal supervision in 1960 compared with 6.14 per cent in 1950. There was a greater use of licensed health workers.

Hemoglobin levels in mothers increased on average although the mean figure of 10.23 grams per 100 ml in 1960 was still below acceptable levels for pregnant women. The increase was attributed to the administration of iron and multi-vitamin pills, and enriched rice. The improvement in maternal care was also reflected in the general decrease in abnormal pregnancies.

There was a considerable increase in the percentage of infants receiving health supervision. Immunization records showed improvement. The height and weight of children from birth to six years of age increased consistently.

The rate of infestation with intestinal parasites did not show the expected improvement despite better sanitary conditions. While the provision of toilets might be expected to have an effect on parasitism, many of the young children defecate indiscriminately and have not learned sufficient hygiene to avoid infestation with worms. The "increase" in hookworm infestation could have been due in part to the improvement in the skills of the laboratory technicians. With ten years of practice, they would be less likely to fail to detect parasitic ova in the stools in 1960 than in 1950.

It is claimed that there was a significant increase in the nutritional status of the population as judged by a decrease in clinical signs. The reporting of these signs is notoriously subjective however and influenced by observer bias. Objective support of the improvement was provided by an increase in urinary riboflavin excretion. This confirmed clinical observations that riboflavin deficiency was less prevalent.

The dental survey showed that there had been in increase in the percentage of school children with one or more teeth decayed, missing, or filled (DMF). This was despite the increase in dental health care and education. It is believed that the urbanization of Novaliches introduced more soft foods, sweets, and candies that facilitated the development of dental caries.

The utilization of health resources had undoubtedly increased and was attributed to the education program, the availability of the resources, and their acceptance by the population.

The completeness of birth registration is important because under-reporting of births gives an inflated *infantile mortality rate* (see page 367).

In 1950, 40.5 per cent of births were not registered. At this level of under-reporting, the *infant mortality rate* was 181.5 per thousand live births while the actual *infant mortality rate* after correction would be 75.4 per thousand.

Other indices of change may be observed in health projects. These may include improvements in general standards of housing and increases in personnel operating in the area in response to public demand. The influx of voluntary agencies, citizen groups, and commerce, may all be positive signs of progress. However, their presence only adds to the problems of evaluating the contribution of the health-promoting components to the project.

A study of the *acceptors* and *rejectors* of health services showed that the *acceptors* belonged to the higher socio-economic groups. They had children in school, and their incomes had increased during the decade. They had more married children and came from larger sized families. They lived near health centers and were conscious of their community problems; they could identify community leaders. The *rejectors*, on the other hand, represented a hard core that lived either in remote or isolated places, or who felt far removed from community activities. They probably had little incentive to live better lives.

The evaluation of the Novaliches project shows that improvements can be brought about although it is not possible to say why they took place. The evaluation of projects has other advantages for it identifies characteristics of people who may accept health services. Evaluation also points out persons requiring some change in their mental, physical, or health environment before they can be expected to turn into acceptors of modern health practices.

Perhaps one of the most important aspects of evaluation is a component that tells the program executive, and administrator, the deficiencies of the service, and to whom it is inaccesible and unacceptable.

Evaluation of applied nutrition programs

An evaluation of applied nutrition programs should refer to the original objectives of the program and to see if the objectives are being achieved. It should provide information that may indicate whether modification to the objectives and *modus operandi*, are required. In addition, evaluation should verify whether the methodology and techniques are adequate for the objectives. Evaluation may also disclose changes in behavior of the community and indicate possibilities for further community participation. Above all, an evaluation tends to restimulate interest in the project.

The process involves survey techniques and it requires, therefore, accurate information and standards that can be used to measure change. In order to gather information, instruments, personnel, funds, and an administrative machine are required. Many projects fail to be effective because they are not evaluated; in many situations evaluation is not carried out because of a lack of funds, expertise or administration.

It is important that evaluation should be "built-in" to the project from the beginning. Participating staff should expect the project to be evaluated, but it is important to insure that it is never considered as a monitoring device, or a means of control.

Three possible approaches have been suggested, depending on costs, time, and staff.[82]

In areas where government services are functioning well and are backed by institutes and universities, a systematic and scientific evaluation should be possible. Where government services are still in the stage of development, evaluation may have to be limited to spot checks and sample surveys. Where health, education, and agriculture are largely rudimentary, evaluation may require the use of visiting experts.

When evaluation is built into a project, the collection of baseline data should include descriptions and indices that might be re-evaluated after an appropriate period of time. Usually an interval of five years or more would elapse between initiating the project and evaluating it. Much of the information would be obtained during the epidemiological evaluation of the nutritional status of the community as described in Chapter 5.

Evaluation may be directed to three aspects of applied nutrition programs. The first is the input of effort and resources. The second is the process and organization of the work program. The third is the output of the program.

Input of effort This is assessed by recording and analyzing changes in administration, investment services, and staff organization. Indicators of change may include increases in budgetary provision for training and education of the public. Opportunities for the public to be exposed to education and training may be measured through an examination of educational services offered through agriculture extension, maternal and child health programs, schools, and the mass media. An appraisal of the numbers and function of the staff may show how much time is actually spent in educational activities. The degree of coverage of the program may be estimated from the numbers of the population served by the services. The impact of the program on government policies also may be measured by noting if all, or part, of the program is being implemented elsewhere.

16*

The process Evaluation of the process of organizing and carrying out the work program involves the assessment of accomplishments of tasks, or changes in the mode of operation of the participants in the program. It may be possible to measure the impact of the education process by examining attendance figures at non-compulsory classes, or by noting the introduction of voluntary groups, or clubs, that are centered around nutrition activities. Changes in agricultural, horticultural, and domestic practices, may also be measured.

It may be possible for example, to note changes in desirable agricultural practices. These may include tie ridging, the increased use of draft animals, small animal breeding, or the presence of fish ponds in an area where these were formerly unknown. Similarly, horticultural indicators may be measured including the planting of varieties resistant to adverse climatic conditions or the cultivation of vegetables that have superior nutritive qualities. The use of the garden as a teaching medium may be noted. Similarly, an indication of progress in the process of education may be obtained from increases in the numbers of persons trained, increases in the number of classes offered, and the number of community participants.

The effects of the program on health may be judged by examining specific death rates, morbidity and mortality experiences, and changes in the prevalence of protein calorie deficiencies. This last effect may be evaluated either from clinical examination or from the *malnutrition score* (see page 435).

A summary of the indicators used for evaluating health is given in Table 97. Further details of the methodology of measurement of these indicators are given in Chapter 5.

The output of the program Changes in nutrition consciousness represent a sequence of events which may lead from an understanding of a problem and recognition of harmful practices, through a series of changes in attitudes or behavior to adoption of new beneficial habits or the abandonment of harmful practices. It may be possible to test public recognition or knowledge of a known nutritive problem. Changes in attitudes and modification of eating practices can be determined from an appraisal of food and nutrient intake. New behavior may be noted and there may be positive indices of a beneficial change having taken place within the group. New innovations such as the cooperative ownership of an oil seed press that produces oil for the community and pressed cake for animal feed, the curing of fish in areas where protein calorie malnutrition was formerly prevalent, can be taken as positive measures. Although they do not guarantee that the infant

Table 97   Indices and measurements for evaluation of applied nutrition programs

Index	
Vital Statistics	Still birth rates,
	Perinatal and neonatal mortality rates,
	Incidence of birth defects
	Infant mortality rates
	Death rate in children 1–4 years
	Second year mortality rate
	Wills Waterlow Index
	Specific death rates from malnutrition
	Specific mortality rates from infections and diarrhea
Prevalence of Protein-Calorie	
Malnutrition	Weight for age and malnutrition score
	Weight for length
	Height for age
	Skinfold thickness
	Arm circumference
	Head and chest circumference
	Biochemical tests—hemoglobin levels
	—serum proteins
	—amino acid patterns
	—serum transferrin
	—urinary excretion of nutrients and metabolites
	—nutrient levels in tissues and tissue fluids

at risk will receive any more high grade protein, at least they are helping to increase its availability.

The indices for evaluation are frequently subjective; further difficulties in the scientific evaluation of programs arise because of the presence of extraneous factors. It may be quite impossible to estimate how much of the observed change is due to the intervention of the program. Scientifically it may be essential to have two separate experimental and control groups. The latter might be expected to show how much progress can be achieved without intervention. One of the criteria for comparative studies of two such groups is that they should be comparable in size and population characteristics, economic, social, and cultural characteristics. In practice it is virtually impossible to "control" applied nutrition programs.

In the meantime, a positive attitude toward evaluation, careful planning, and a methodical approach may succeed in producing data which will help administrators to decide whether the program should be continued or not. The evaluation of the *Bayambang Applied Nutrition Program* in the Philippines was considered so successful that similar projects were encouraged elsewhere in the islands. Some of the conclusions were however, unexpected. For example, the provision of vitamin and mineral supplements and deworming did not give evidence of improved growth.

It had been assumed that the presence of maternal and child health services were taking care of infant problems. This was not the case however, for the services were very much diluted by the size of the population and the separation of the *barrios*. The infant and toddler feeding program helped to fill the gap in the services.

The *applied nutrition program* was found to be very effective in offering instruction in 'basic MCH' given by school teachers and *barrio* workers associated with the project. This alone is probably a justification for community orientated programs since once a health problem is defined and accepted by the public, their involvement in its solution is not only more probable, but it may well lead to the recognition of other health problems. The Philippine experience provides further support for the suggestion made earlier in this chapter concerning the future for community nutrition programs. The development of community programs probably rests on the establishment of local community nutrition committees rather than on top level program intervention by central government agencies.

The education components of the Bayambang project was an undoubted success. Response to education was recorded in staff participating in the program and also at the grass roots level in the community.

The *Bayambang applied nutrition program* was a pilot program designed, in part, to examine the feasibility of using similar projects elsewhere in the Philippines and it has been evaluated as successful. To be realistic it must be remembered that the nutrition problems in the Philippines are enormous and it will take many thousand *applied nutrition projects* to make an impact on the health of the Filipinos. The *applied nutrition program* should not be considered an answer to national nutrition problems but one of the tools that may be used by nutritionists to bring about changes in food habits. This is the ultimate aim of all nutrition programs and services. The provision of information and education in nutrition is often assumed to be the initial step in a series of events that are assumed to end in change. The inadequacies of evaluation and the failure to evaluate nutrition programs and services has led to complacency over the effectiveness of nutrition education. Changes in food habits are not the inevitable result of providing information and knowledge. The difficult task of bringing about change is the subject of the next and final chapter.

References

1. Williams, C. D. *Factors in the Ecology of Malnutrition.* Proceedings Western Hemisphere Nutrition Congress, p. 20. American Medical Association, Chicago, 1966.

2. Folling, A. "Über Ausscheidung von Phenylbrenztraubensäure in den Harn als Stoffwechselanomalie in Verbindung mit Imezillitat." *Hoppe Seyler Z. Physiol. Chem.* **227**: 169, 1934.

3. Guthrie, R., Susi, A. "A Simple Phenylalanine Method for Detecting Phenylketonuria in Large Populations of Newborn Infants." *Pediatrics* **32**: 338, 1963.

4. Guthrie, R., Whitney, S. *Phenylketonuria Detection in the Newborn Infant as a Routine Hospital Procedure.* Childrens Bureau Publication No. 419, Washington, D. C. 1964.

5. Massachusetts Department of Health. "Screening Program for Phenylketonuria and Other Inborn Errors of Metabolism." *New Eng. J. Med.* **273**: 109, 1965.

6. President of the United States. *White House Conference on Food Nutrition and Health.* Final Report, p. 8. Washington, D. C. 1969.

7. Bray, H. "The Costs of Malnutrition." *Appalachia* **2**:6, 1969.

8. Awan, A. H. "The System of Local Health Services in Rural Pakistan" Public Health Association of Pakistan, Lahore, 1969.

9. Barraclough, S. Papers on Agrarian Reform, No. 2. Instituto de Capacitacion e investigacion en reforma agraria.

10. Latham, M. C. "Some Observations Relating to Applied Nutrition Projects Supported by the U. N. Agencies." *Nutr. Rev.* **25**: 193, 1967.

11. King, M. (ed.) *Medical Care in Developing Countries.* Nairobi: Oxford University Press, 1966.

12. Fendall, N. R. E. "Planning Health Services in Developing Countries." *Pub. Hlth. Rep.* **78**: 977, 1963.

13. "Organization of M. C. H. in Developing Regions." *J. Trop. Ped.* Vol. **12**, 1966 and Vol. **13**, 1967.

14. Gomez, F., Galvan, R., Cravioto, J., Frenk, S. "Malnutrition in Infancy and Childhood, with Special Reference to Kwashiorkor." *Advances in Pediatrics.* **7**: 131, 1955. New York: The Yearbook Publishers, 1955.

15. Hill, M. M. "Nutrition Committees and Nutrition Education." *J. Nutr. Educ.* **1**: 14, 1969.

16. Weinerman, E. R. *Social Medicine in Eastern Europe*, p. 29. Harvard University Press, 1969.

17. Davis, H. P. Sharing Our Bounty. In *Food.* The Yearbook of Agriculture, p. 681. Washington, D. C.: U. S. Government Printing Office, 1959.

18. Vanneman, S. C. School Lunch to Food Stamp: America Cares for its Hungry. In *Food for Us All.* Yearbook of Agriculture, p. 69. Washington, D. C.: U. S. Government Printing Office, 1969.

19. Harris, R. S. "Attitudes and Approaches to Supplementation of Foods With Nutrients." *J. Ag. Food Chem.* **16**: 149, 1968.

20. LeBovit, C. "U. S. Diets and Enrichment." *J. Ag. Food Chem.* **16**: 153, 1968.

21. Howe, E. E., Jansen, G. R., Gilfillan, E. W. "Amino Acid Supplementation of Cereal Grain as Related to the World Food Supply." *Amer. J. Clin Nutr.* **16**:315, 1965.

22. Hegsted, D. M. "Amino Acid Fortification and the Protein Problem." *Amer. J. Clin. Nutr.* **21**: 688, 1968.

23. "Food Additives." *The Lancet* **2**: 361, 1969.
24. Sanders, H. J. "Food Additives," *Chemical and Engineering News*. October 1966.
25. Boyd, E. M., Stefec, J. "Dietary Protein and Pesticide Toxicity: With Particular Reference to Endrin." *Canad. Med. Ass. J.* **101**: 335, 1969.
26. Guthrie, R., Susi, A. "A Simple Phenylalanine Method for Detecting Phenylketonuria in Large Populations of Newborn Infants." *Pediatrics* **32**: 338, 1963.
27. Levy, H. L., Karolkewicz, V., Houghton, S. A., MacCready, R. "Screening the 'Normal' Population in Massachusetts for Phenylketonuria." *New Eng. J. Med.* **282**: 1455, 1970.
28. Hammar, S. L. "The Role of the Nutritionist in an Adolescent Clinic." *Children* **13**: 217, 1966.
29. McMurray, G. L. "Project Teen Aid: A Community Action Approach to Services for Pregnant Unmarried Teen-Agers." *Amer. J. Public Health* **58**: 1848, 1968.
30. Pell, S., D'Alonzo, C. A. "Acute Myocardial Infarction in a Large Industrial Population." *J. Amer. Med. Ass.* **185**: 831, 1963.
31. Latham, M. C., Robson, J. R. K. "A Trial to Evaluate the Benefit of Different Protein Rich Foods to African School Children." *Nutr. Dieta.* **7**: 28, 1965.
32. Baertl, J. M., Morales, E., Verastegui, G., Graham, G. G. "Diet Supplementation of Entire Communities." *Amer. J. Clin. Nutr.* **23**: 707, 1970.
33. Figueria, F., Mendonca, S., Rocha, J., Azevedo, M., Bunce, G. E., Reynolds, J. W. "Absorption of Vitamin A by Infants Receiving Fat-Free or Fat-Containing Dried Skim Milk Formulas." *Amer. J. Clin. Nutr.* **22**: 588, 1969.
34. Srikantia, S. G., Reddy, V. "Effect of a Single Massive Dose of Vitamin A on Serum and Liver Levels of the Vitamin." *Amer. J. Clin. Nutr.* **23**: 114, 1970.
35. Swaminathan, M. C., Sushella, T. P., Thimmayamma, B. V. S. "Field Prophylactic Trial With a Single Oral Massive Dose of Vitamin A." *Amer. J. Clin. Nutr.* **23**:119,1970.
36. Lian, O. K., Tie, L. Y., Rose, C. S., Prawiranegara, D., Gyorgy, P. "Red Palm Oil in the Prevention of Vitamin A Deficiency." *Paediatrica Indonesia* **8**: 192, 1968.
37. Kevany, J., Chopra, J. G. "The Use of Iodized Oil in Goiter Prevention." *Amer. J. Public Health* **60**: 919, 1970.
38. Committee on Maternal Nutrition, Food and Nutrition Board. National Research Council. "Maternal Nutrition and the Course of Pregnancy." National Academy of Sciences, Washington, D. C., 1970.
39. Chaudhuri, S. K. "Relationship of Protein-Calorie Malnutrition with Toxemia of Pregnancy." *Amer. J. Obstet. Gynecol.* **107**: 33, 1970.
40. Pike, R. L., Gursky, D. S. "Further Evidence of Deleterious Effects Produced by Sodium Restriction During Pregnancy." *Amer. J. Clin. Nutr.* **23**: 883, 1970.
41. Taggart, N. R., Holliday, R. M., Billewicz, W. Z., Hytten, F. E., Thomson, A. M. "Changes in Skinfolds During Pregnancy." *Brit. J. Nutr.* **21**: 439, 1967.
42. Bonnar, J., Goldberg, A., Smith, J. A. "Do Pregnant Women Take Their Iron?" *The Lancet* **1**: 457, 1969.
43. Thomson, A. M., Hytten, F. E., Billewicz, W. Z. "The Energy Cost of Human Lactation." *Brit. J. Nutr.* **24**: 565, 1970.
44. Raynaud, A. Morphogenesis of the Mammary Gland. In *Milk: The Mammary Gland and Its Secretion*, p. 11. Eds. Kon, S. K., Cowie, A. T. New York: Academic Press, 1961.
45. Hirsch, J., Knittle, J. L. "Cellularity of Obese and Nonobese Human Adipose Tissue." Fed. Proc. **29**: 1516, 1970.

46. Mayer, J. *Overweight Causes, Cost* and *Control*, p. 160, Prentice Hall, 1968.
47. Lawlor, T., Wells, D. G. "Metabolic Hazards of Fasting." *Amer. J. Clin. Nutr.* **22**: 1142, 1969.
48. Bloom, W. L., Eidex, M. F. "The Comparison of Energy Expenditure in the Obese and Lean." *Metabolism* **16**: 685, 1968.
49. Stunkard, A. J. "Environment and Obesity: Recent Advances in Our Understanding of Regulation of Food Intake in Man." *Fed. Proc.* **27**: 1367, 1968.
50. Schachter, S., Gross, L. P. "Manipulated Time and Eating Behavior." *J. Personality and Soc. Psychology*, **10**: 98, 1968.
51. Schachter, S. "Obesity and Eating." *Science*, **161**: 751, 1968.
52. Cornell Conferences on Therapy. "The Management of Obesity." *New York State J. Medicine* **58**: 79, 1958.
53. Shipman, W. G., Plesset, M. R. "Predicting the Outcome for Obese Dieters." *J. Amer. Diet. Ass.* **42**: 383, 1963.
54. Stuart, R. B. "Behavioral Control of Overeating." *Behav. Res. and Ther.* **5**: 357, 1967.
55. Penick, S. B., Filion, R., Fox, S., Stunkard, A. J. Behavior Modification in the Treatment of Obesity. Annual Meeting, American Psychosomatic Society, March 1970.
56. Sherwood, S. "Gerontology and the Sociology of Food and Eating." *Aging and Human Development* **1**: 61, 1970.
57. Shock, N. "Physiological Aspects of Aging." *J. Amer. Diet. Ass.* **56**: 491, 1970.
58. Pearson, R. C. M. "Feeding the Elderly in Their Own Homes: Meeting the Need." *Proc. Nutr. Soc.* **27**:37, 1968.
59. "Meals Plus Offered by Detroit Project." *Aging*, No. 184–185, Feb.–Mar. 1970, p. 18.
60. Research Committee of the Medical Research Council. "Controlled Trial of Soya-Bean Oil in Myocardial Infarction." *The Lancet* **2**: 693, 1968.
61. Dayton, S., Pearce, M. L., Goldman, H., Harnish, A., Plotkin, D., Schickman, M., Winfield, M., Zager, A., Dixon, W. "Controlled Trial of a Diet High in Unsaturated Fat for Prevention of Atherosclerotic Complications." *The Lancet* **2**: 1060, 1968.
62. The National Diet-Heart Study, Final Report. *Circulation* **37**: Supplement No. 1, 1968.
63. Bengoa, J. M. "Nutrition Rehabilitation Centers." *J. Trop. Ped.* **13**: 169, 1967.
64. Garrow, J. S. "Treatment of Malnutrition." *The Lancet* **2**: 324, 1969.
65. Garrow, J. S., Smith, R., Ward, E. *Electrolyte Balance in Severe Infantile Malnutrition*. London: Pergamon Press, 1968.
66. Wharton, B. A., Jelliffe, D. B., Stanfield, J. P. "Do We Know How to Treat Kwashiorkor." *J. Pediat.* **72**: 721, 1968.
67. Adams, E. B. "Anemia Associated with Kwashiorkor." *Amer. J. Clin. Nutr.* **22**: 1634, 1969.
68. Robson, J. R. K. "The Operation and Function of Malwards." Report to the World Health Organization Western Pacific Regional Office, Manila 1970.
69. Beghin, I. D. "Nutritional Rehabilitation Centers in Latin America: A Critical Assessment." *Amer. J. Clin. Nutr.* **23**: 1412, 1970.
70. Morley, D., Bicknell, J., Woodland, M. "Factors Influencing the Growth and Nutritional Status of Infants and Young Children in a Nigerian Village." *Trans. Roy. Soc. Trop Med. Hyg.* **62**: 164, 1968.
71. Gokulunathan, K. S. "Nutrition Clinics and Child Care Programs." *Clin. Pediat.* **8**: 502, 1969.

72. Wilkinson, J. L. "Children in Hospital in Sierra Leone: A Survey of 10,000 Admissions." *Trans. Roy. Soc. Trop. Med. Hyg.* **63**: 263, 1969.

73. Bailey, K. V. Report of a Pilot Project in Applied Nutrition in Bayambang, Pangasinan, Philippines. World Health Organization, Regional Office for the Western Pacific, Manila, 1966.

74. A Strategy for Plenty: The Indicative World Plan for Agricultural Development. World Food Problems No. 11, F. A. O. Rome 1970.

75. Pirie, N. W. "Complementary Ways of Meeting the World's Protein Need." *Proc. Nutr. Soc.* **28**: 255, 1969.

76. FAO/WHO/UNICEF Protein Advisory Group United Nations, PAG Bulletin No. 9, New York 1970.

77. Becroft, T., Bailey, K. V. "Supplementary Feeding Trial in New Guinea Highland Infants." *J. Trop. Pediat.* **11**: 28, 1965.

78. Bolan, T. D., Davis, A. E. "Asian Lactose Intolerance and Its Relation to Intake of Lactose." *Nature* **222**: 382, 1969.

79. "Lactose Deficiency in Thailand." *Nutr. Rev.* **27**: 278, 1969

80. Browe, J. H. "Evaluation of a Nutrition Program." *J. Amer. Diet. Ass.* **31**: 895, 1955.

81. Tiglao, T. V. "Health Practices in a Rural Community." Community Development Research Council. University of the Philippines, Quezon City, 1968.

82. "Methods of Planning and Evaluation in Applied Nutrition Programs." World Health Organization, Tech. Report Series No. 340, WHO, Geneva, 1966.

CHAPTER 7

Food Habits: Cultural Determinants and Methodology of Change

In the discussion that follows, the term "change" is used as a concept that includes all the processes involved in bringing about an alteration in food habits.

Food habits

When an individual is found to have a nutritional problem, correcting the situation should include not only the therapeutic aspect of supplying the nutrients needed to alter the disease state but also the preventive aspect of altering the environment that gave rise to the problem. For example, a child with protein calorie malnutrition requires specific treatment for the condition. However, if the factors which gave rise to the condition, such as a lack of knowledge on the relationship between food and health, are not altered, relapse is inevitable. The diet is part of the environment of malnutrition and the suggestions for change must be as carefully chosen as the prescription of specific nutrients which are needed to correct the dietary deficiency. The prescribed diet must be nutritious yet its provision should not exceed the economic resources of the family, and it must be based on more than the supposition that the food is a carrier of nutrients. Nutrients are found in food but people seldom choose a food for the nutrient value alone. Food is eaten to satisfy hunger, for pleasure and comfort. In some instances, adding a locally available food to the diet or providing a new food product that has an ideal nutrient content may relieve a nutritional problem, but access to such a food cannot assure its inclusion in the diet. The adoption or rejection of the suggestion will depend upon the cultural definition of food and the perceived advantage of the change within the society where the nutritional problem developed.

A change in food habits must be made if a nutritional problem is to be eliminated rather than temporarily alleviated. In order to bring about change, it is necessary first to understand the economic, social, and cultural factors which influence dietary patterns, food intake, and thus, nutritional status. The cause as well as the result of inadequate intake must be considered. A thorough understanding of the cause will provide a valid basis for programs designed to bring about change.

Change must be in a specific direction and it inevitably involves the diffusion of knowledge about food, nutrients, and the function of nutrients in the body. The propagation of nutrition information is vitally important if habits are to be changed in a beneficial direction.

Information is being imparted to the public in a number of ways and situations. For example, information is offered to patients by the medical, nursing, and dental professions; it is also offered by dietitians, or nutritionists, as a therapeutic or preventive measure.

The mass media of radio, television, newspapers, and magazines are constantly trying to change food habits by advertising specific food products. Whether the appeal is based on nutrient or caloric value, taste, status, or novelty, its intention is to induce change in the food intake that will insure the inclusion of a specific product in the diet. Finally, there are the informal channels of communication through friends, relatives, and neighbors that provide information and opinions on food and nutrition.

The sources of information may be limited or many and diverse but all represent a form of dictated change. The supposition, often unstated, is that the person who adopts these changes will be a more admirable or healthy person than one who does not respond.

While an individual is exposed to specific suggestions for changes in his diet, he is also exposed to the influence of general trends in food consumption. In the past few decades, many changes have taken place in the broad patterns of food consumption in most parts of the world.

There are new foods such as soft drinks and dessert toppings; old foods in a new form such as the processed cheese spreads and peanut butter; and many new prepared, ready-to-eat foods. In the United States a nationwide survey indicated an increase in use and expenditure on convenience foods.[1] Expenditures on selected convenience foods averaged $ 1.84 per person per week in 1955; the figure rose to $ 2.47 in 1965. These foods represented twenty-seven per cent of the total expenditure for purchased food in 1955 and thirty per cent in 1965. During this same period, the pattern of consumption of food groups varied. The consumption of foods included in the meat group (meat, poultry, fish, eggs, dry beans, dry peas, and nuts) increased from 5.2 pounds per person per week to 5.7 pounds. The use of other major groups of food decreased; the milk group from 9.6 to 8.8 pounds, the vegetable and fruit group from 9.9 to 9.1 pounds, and the bread and cereal group from 2.8 to 2.6 pounds. The use of fats and oils, sugars and sweets remained about the same by weight. While the nature of the change is readily described, it is difficult to isolate any one causal factor that has brought about the change.

Alterations in food habits in the United States have occurred concurrently with general shifts in the style of living. An increasing number of families live in urban centers and the opportunity for the home production of food has decreased. Women are employed outside the home, consequently the time available for shopping and preparation of food is less. Not eating at home is even more convenient and the increase in the number of franchise restaurants specializing in inexpensive meals is a reflection of that habit. In this age of rapid communication and transportation, the effect of science and technology on dietary habits is evident not only in the United States but in all parts of the world. Coca Cola, granulated sugar and white flour are products of food technology that can be found in parts of the world far from the place of manufacture. In the production of butter, skim milk is a by-product and was fed to pigs before methods of dehydration were perfected. Now dry skim milk in plastic packages is sent routinely to remote areas of the world. Refrigerators represent modern technology in the villages of Africa and offer the owners an opportunity to alter their traditional methods of food buying and consumption. Proprietary infant formulae made in the United states, Holland, and England are found in the most remote villages and offer an alternative to breast feeding.

Food habits change as the products of technology become available, but the direction of change does not necessarily result in the improvement of nutritional status. The problem appears to be one of implementing change that will have beneficial effects in the midst of a dynamic world that produces random changes in dietary patterns which may, or may not, be beneficial.

Mead suggested that the question to be asked is not "How do you change food habits?" but "How are food habits changed?"[2] We need to know how food habits are established: how the child learns to eat and how much; how learning about food is reinforced by the social and economic aspects of community life; whether people accept scientific knowledge and in what form; how an eating pattern can be modified to fit present-day nutritional knowledge and yet be flexible enough to change when necessary; and finally, what can be learned from past experience that will guide us in our efforts to improve food habits?

The food habits of an individual reflect a lifetime of experience with food. They represent the result of receiving, classifying, and collating in-

formation and its application to an eating pattern that is feasible and preferable under prevailing living conditions and economic means. Many factors
influence the daily choice of food. An understanding of the relative effect
of these factors upon the individual or family is essential to the nutrition
educator who wishes to be an effective change agent.

How food habits are established

Determinants of food habits

Many investigators have been concerned with the identification of factors
that operate in the decision-making process and which result in the food
choices of individuals and households. Any food that is eaten is a symbol
of a decision made in response to a physiological or psychological need.
How is that decision made? A household is often defined as those individuals who eat from the same cooking pot. Does a meal represent a group
decision, or does the person who prepared the food decide what is to be
included in the meal? One analysis of the situation suggests that food comes
to the table by channels controlled by a "gatekeeper". Usually this is the
housewife, who defines what is "food", and selects items according to
her values which may include taste, status, cost, and health.[3]

Availability, price, familiarity, time for preparation, and other factors
play a part in the decision-making process. It should be kept in mind,
however, that these factors do not necessarily operate alone, or one-by-one,
but represent relative weightings in the mind of the individual. It is quite
obvious that cost may be outweighed by convenience and it is possible
that knowledge of the nutrient value may be overridden by cultural preference
or prejudice. The economic advantage of a food appears to be one of the
strong factors that influence food choices, yet there are examples where
this is clearly not the most important factor. In order to celebrate a wedding
or religious holiday, the poorest family will often borrow money rather
than mar the occasion with a culturally unsuitable food. Even though
horse meat may be inexpensive, prejudice prevents many individuals from
recognizing it as food for humans. There are factors which influence food
habits, but we do not know which factors carry the strongest weight in any
specific situation, nor do we know how these factors operate in conjunction
to each other. Some of these individual influences and their interrelationships will be discussed in further detail.

Familiarity Previous experience is one of the strong influences upon individual dietary choices. Experience within the home teaches the child what is

considered edible and even when to eat it. When the terms "likes" and "dislikes" are used, they refer to judgements made on the basis of past experience. Evaluation may be founded not upon personal reaction but upon those of other family members or friends.

In a study designed to explore the eating behavior of preschool children of the North Central Region of the United States, mothers were asked about the fruit and vegetable preferences of their offspring.[4] Eighteen per cent of the children who had been given vegetables were reported to dislike these foods; only three per cent of the children who had been given fruits reported dislikes or refusals. Although distaste for vegetables tended to be associated more with the dislikes of the father than the dislikes of the mother, they were even more closely related to the dislikes of older siblings, particularly older brothers.

In another group of children of similar age and geographic location, the offspring generally agreed with the likes and dislikes of their parents.[5] The highest correlation between the attitudes of children and their parents was on the preference for vegetables, particularly those least liked by the children.

Specific vegetables are often listed as food items that are disliked. This may be partially due to the wide variety of foods classed under the general heading of vegetables. The variety of meats is much less, consequently there is a greater chance of them becoming known and therefore acceptable. When a wider variety of vegetables is available, there is more opportunity for children to encounter one that is unfamiliar. In the case of foods, unfamiliarity rather than familiarity seems to breed contempt.

The failure of people to accept a new food is often attributed to un-acquaintance. Improved varieties of wheat were promoted by the Community Development Projects in Uttar Pradash in India.[6] The new varieties had a higher yield, lower cost with higher nutrient content, high disease and drought resistant properties, and good marketability. Despite these ad-vantages, the new varieties were not initially accepted as a replacement for the familiar wheat because the new food had a strange color, flat taste, and the women found it difficult to use as flour. Use of one variety of wheat had led to the consumers developing a set of standards for wheat and the new variety did not conform to these. The new variety was initially rejected, but later it gained acceptance as consumers adjusted their standards.

Using familiarity as a basis for changing food habits proved successful in a feeding program in East Africa.[7] In a school feeding trial, acceptance of protein-rich supplementary foods was one criterion used to evaluate the potential of various foods as a mid-day snack. The several products which were tested included ground nut flour preparations, maize meal and skimmed milk mixtures, meat powder, and a defatted soya bean flour made into a gruel. This last product was the most acceptable although it was a new food product. All the other commodities were known and accepted as food sources in other forms, but they were virtually unknown as presented to the school children. The soya bean gruel was the consistency and color of their own maize staple, and it had an aroma and taste of beans, a food familiar to them. In the other cases, a strange color (ground nut flour), an unfamiliar taste (dried skimmed milk and maize mixture) or too watery consistency (meat powder) seemed to adversely affect the acceptability.

One of the elements in familiarity may be the conditions under which the food was introduced. In a study of three to four year old children in the United States, twenty-three per cent of the mothers used foods as rewards for good behavior and ten per cent used food deprivation as punishment.[8] Reward foods included baked goods and desserts (75 per cent), sweets (39 per cent), and fruit (32 per cent). Although sweets were used as a reward, the mothers reported that this was the only type of food that created concern when there was overconsumption.

Foods classified by mothers as "pleasure foods", such as candy, sweet foods, or carbonated beverages, are often used as a reward for good behavior. The amount of money spent by adults and adolescents for candy, sweet foods, and soft drinks may be due largely to the associations formed in the early years of life. If these foods were used as rewards, they are familiar and have positive connotations.

Income   This is one of the most reliable indicators of dietary adequacy. While adequate income does not guarantee the family a nutritionally adequate diet, nutrient needs must be met by foods purchased or obtained from other sources. Usually families in the United States with a low income cannot spend more than one-third or one-fourth of their income on food and meet other basic needs for shelter and clothing. Three times the cost of a minimal, nutritionally adequate diet is generally accepted as the poverty level index for eligibility to many poverty programs but the cost of the diet varies according to local retail prices.

Many foods, by reason of their price, are not available to the consumer with a limited budget. The concept of a diet for the poor and a diet for the rich may be unacceptable to democratic ideals but the condition nevertheless exists. Foods that are in short supply and conform to the society's concept of "good" foods, command a high market price. The family with a small amount of money for food is interested in items that are cheap and have the property of filling the belly and giving a feeling of satiety. Many of these foods not only help to prevent hunger but they are also good energy sources; unfortunately their contribution of protein is often unsatisfactory.

The development of specific food habits from the condition of poverty is not well documented. In general, low income is correlated with nutrient inadequacy and high carbohydrate consumption.[1] Protein-rich foods are usually higher in price than foods that are mainly carbohydrate. In a sample of midwestern families, low-income households ate more white potatoes and less fruit than high-income families, a practice directly related to the retail cost of the food products.[5]

The cost of a food item is often affected by the place where it was purchased. In the poverty areas of Omaha, Nebraska, neighborhood stores were abundant in number and widely distributed but they had poorer standards of hygiene and charged higher prices; quality items, when available, cost more.[9] On the average, chain stores provided lower prices and offered better quality and standards of hygiene. The impoverished consumer has little control over where he spends his money. On a limited income, there may be no money to hire someone to care for the children, no car, no bus or taxi fare-in short, no freedom. They are fenced into a small geographic purchasing area by economic and psychological barriers, a situation true for both the rural and the metropolitan poor. "Poor is buying in the neighborhood at whatever the prices happen to be."[10]

It seems reasonable to assume that within the low-income category, the money available for food dictates the degree of consideration given to other factors that influence food consumption. Low-income families in Mississippi who qualified to receive commodity foods through the United States Department of Agriculture program, did not use all that were available.[11] Bulgour, rolled wheat, grits, split peas and cornmeal were used infrequently. The reasons why these foods were unpopular were not explored but the finding suggests that acceptance does not necessarily follow supply even within economic restrictions.

There may be a minimal level below which supply or availability is the determining factor in acceptance, but that level may be one step removed from starvation. When the alternative is hunger, a food may be eaten without real acceptance. True acceptance of a product as food would be evident if the food item remains as a part of the diet after the emergency passes.

An interesting reversal of the relationship between income and food consumption is seen in the case of *soul foods*. Soul foods currently have an ethnic connotation and they are popular in all income levels in both the northern and southern regions of the United States. The term refers to the type of food, such as sweet potatoes, turnip or collard greens, cornbread, grits, and pork products, and the method of preparation. Fried ham with red eye gravy, greens stewed with meat, cornbread, and sweet potato pie are the ingredients for a typical soul food meal. These foods were originally simple foods that were inexpensive or free to the low-income residents of the southern United States. The share-croppers or small farm operators could raise pigs, grow corn, and gather greens that required little if any cultivation. These foods are no longer inexpensive, but taste preferences have been established and have persisted despite a change in the cost advantage.

Preparation time   The time required to prepare food is often a major point of consideration in the meal planning done by the housewife. Foods requiring little preparation in the home have gained in popularity in the past few years. Convenience sells in the food market as it does elsewhere.

Convenience foods is a new term that has arisen in recent years. It is applied to foods partly processed or prepared before sale. This reduces the time that has to be spent on its preparation in the home.

According to a nationwide food consumption survey in the United States, in the spring of 1965 three of ten food dollars were spent on convenience foods.[12] In comparison to the spending in 1955, there was an increase in the consumption of fresh and commercial fruit juices, canned and condensed soups, dehydrated soups, ready-to-eat breakfast cereals, and powders which form the basis of fruit drinks and instant coffee. The proportionate increase in use of convenience foods was greater in low-income groups than in higher-income households. The amount of money expended on convenience foods in samples of low-income households increased by 47 per cent. This compares with an average of 34 per cent for all households and an increase of 28 per cent for high-income households. At the end of the ten year period, there was less differentiation between urban and rural areas and different regions of the United States than there was at the beginning of the period.

The influence of preparation time on food habits is illustrated by a study of American Negroes.[13] During the past six decades, many Negro Americans have exchanged a rural southern environment for one in the urban north. The basic diet has undergone little change, although compensatory changes in the serving time and terminology of meals have been made. The traditional breakfast often consisted of meats, rice, biscuits, potatoes, and a beverage. This pattern continued for an average of 18 months in the new environment.

The main meal traditionally was eaten in midafternoon and called dinner. It consisted of boiled vegetables seasoned with meat and accompanied by cornbread, potatoes, a beverage, and an occasional dessert. In the new urban environment breakfast consists of eggs, hot biscuits or bread, and coffee, a much lighter meal than the traditional breakfast. Instead of leftovers from breakfast, the new lunch taken at, or near work, consists of sandwiches, soup, crackers, raw fruits and a fruit drink. The main meal is served in the evening and called supper.

On holidays and weekends, there is a reversion to the traditional breakfast pattern. The contemporary evening meal is a combination of the traditional dinner and breakfast. The change of living pattern has changed the traditional five "boiling days" (weekday meals when the dinner consisted of a heavy boiled dinner) to two or three "boiling days" and two or three "frying days".

The new patterns of food consumption can be attributed to the carry over of previous living conditions as well as the contemporary social situation of American Negroes who are restricted by *de facto* segregation in northern urban areas.

Methods of food preparation change to conform to the demands of modern urban living, but the changes to simplified preparation may in turn generate an influence on family living patterns. The cooperative activities which are part of the many operations involved in the preparation of foods required for a family meal, bring the family members together. With the advent of convenience foods, cooperative activities are no longer needed.[14] The increasing "convenience" of foods may have also a direct effect on social behavior, making individuals in the family less dependent on each other for meals. Shared meals are assumed to be an important aspect of a harmonious society. This concept implies that we should reintroduce an element of rawness into food, requiring a family to exercise a degree of technical and social skill, rather than pursuing convenience, standardization, and efficiency to their ultimate limit. Rather than encouraging the progression to convenient, individually pre-wrapped bites of food, it might be useful to help units of society to coalesce again. This may be achieved by offering "inconvenience" foods which would demand the presence of the whole family to prepare and consume. Steps in this direction might restore a measure of corporate health lost in the pursuit of individual nutrition.

Food conventions and taboos Fine distinctions are made between what is "food" and what is "not food". Some foods are considered fit for animals

17*

but not for man. The remark, "it looks like dog food", leaves no doubt
that the person who uttered the remark neither likes the appearance of the
food in question nor does he consider it fit for consumption. The decision
on whether a food should be consumed may depend on whether the food
is considered "clean" or "unclean". Vegetable peelings or table scraps may
be considered unclean and therefore designated as "animal foods". These
decisions may be quite irrational. Vegetable peelings removed before the
vegetable reaches the serving table may be called "unclean", yet children
are urged to eat the skin of a baked potato because it contains vitamins.
Soybeans and corn are produced specifically for animal feed. The new
simulated meat products made of soy protein may have to overcome the
"food for animals" image that still clings to soy products.

Within the range of foods regarded as "food acceptable to humans",
further distinctions may be recognized. It is not unusual, for example, to
characterize some human groups by their apparent bizarre or unusual
food habits. Even whole nations may be designated as frog eaters, snail
eaters, or dog eaters. The characterizations seldom express envy, but
derision.

Even within the smaller group of the family or religious group, there
may be a further definition of what is "food for me". Particular foods
for holidays or treats may be specified. Within the family, children learn
to feel that the food they eat is part of themselves, and the attitude of other
people toward their food may be construed as personal acceptance or
criticism.

Beliefs   There are many instances of beliefs related to food consumption.
Some of these beliefs are based on religion or health; others may be related
to magic or wish-fulfillment. When sources of food are limited and the
maintenance of life is dependent upon an uncertain supply of food, beliefs
and superstitions can readily develop and govern the distribution and consumption of food. Should the consumption of a food be clearly but in-
explicably related to a health hazard, the regulation of consumption of
that food may be reinforced by its incorporation into a religious or other
belief system.

The classification of foods into categories of "hot" and "cold" has been
observed in different cultures. The concept does not apply to the temperature
of the food but to some innate quality ascribed to the food. In India[15]
and Peru,[16] foods are believed to produce a heating or cooling effect on
the body. The properties are used in the treatment of various illnesses.
In the study of a Peruvian community, thermal categorization of specific

foods was employed primarily as an explanation of illness. Under normal conditions, dietary preferences were relatively free of categorization into hot or cold. Some foods, such as turnip leaves were classified as cold and regarded unfavorably. Although vitamin A deficiency was prevalent, turnip leaves which could have eliminated the deficiency, were not consumed. The study suggests that new foods are classified ambivalently unless some association with health develops. If a new food introduced into the community cannot be classified immediately, it is probable that it will be adopted.

Food beliefs with little scientific basis are not restricted to technologically underdeveloped societies. The use of vitamin pills is an example of a practice that has grown beyond its scientific basis and could be classed as a belief. The realization that vitamins are needed by the body in order to perform certain functions has prompted many people to believe that the more vitamins consumed, the better the results. Mothers who give their infants overdoses of fat-soluble vitamins are motivated by beliefs rather than nutrition knowledge.

Advertisements and packages of breakfast cereals and other foods often feature a central figure in the form of an athlete or folk hero. It is implied that if the product is eaten, the result will not only be satisfaction, but the physical attributes and achievements of the central figure will be duplicated. This belief resembles those of the members of a primitive tribe who eat jaguars, bulls, and stags to make them strong, brave, and swift.

The use of macrobiotic vegetarian diets is based on a belief system which is not substantiated by scientific data, but it is strongly supported by individuals subscribing to the philosophy of Zen macrobiotics.[17] The philosophy includes the belief that disease is caused by an imbalance of Yin and Yang in the body. The balance of Yin and Yang qualities in the body can be altered by eating foods which provide the ideal balance. The ideal proportion is five Yin to one Yang; this is provided by a pure cereal diet of brown rice. Foods are classified according to the predominance of Yin and Yang factors. A range of diets is suggested. Number seven is the easiest, simplest and "wisest" diet; it consists of cereals and a sparing amount of liquid. Diet number one includes cereals, vegetables, soup, animal products and liquid. Some of these regimes may be harmful. For example, a 36-year old woman consumed a diet of pressure-cooked brown rice, salted and sprinkled with sesame seeds, ground oatmeal, cornmeal, buckwheat, bread made from cooked rice and 12 ounces of soup or tea.[18] The diet was followed for eight months. During this period, she lost weight, developed scurvy, and symptoms of folic acid and protein deficiency. The patient suffered a severe physical disability and was near death before she was persuaded to accept hospitalization and medical care.

The potential of the wide variety of dietary beliefs encountered in various societies are far from being understood. It is impossible to proscribe all forms of unusual diets as universally harmful and lacking in benefit. Individuals may attest to the efficacy of a particular diet, but seldom, if ever, are there controlled, objective studies to support or refute the claims. Nutritionists usually find ignorance easier to accept than a belief system than runs counter to their own. Suggestions to supplement the diet within the limitations of the philosophy may be more useful than outright condemnation. Instead of ridiculing beliefs that represent an earnest search for ways to improve health through the diet, an interest in diet and foods should be encouraged and knowledge enlarged.

Nutrition knowledge

Acquisition of nutrition knowledge   Although there is a body of knowledge, developed through systematic investigation which can be labeled "the science of nutrition", there coexists a basic concept of food needs, that may have no scientific foundation. These concepts are found in individuals in the most sophisticated societies and the most primitive tribes. At the simplest level, an individual may know only what foods are "good", safe, and available. A more knowledgeable person may know of some foods which should be eaten during specific stages of the life cycle, or perhaps foods to cure or prevent illness, or he may have opinions on food items for festive occasions.

This latter person has received information on nutrition, although the amount represents a relatively small percentage of the total information theoretically available. Although this knowledge may be limited and sometimes inaccurate, there is, nevertheless, a reservoir of information which influences behavior in choosing and consuming food.

The aim of nutrition education is to bring the nutrition knowledge of each individual to the point where he makes the wisest choice of food within the existing economic limitations. The supplementation of the knowledge of an individual requires not only contact with new information but an understanding of the material. There are a number of potential sources of information; printed material, radio, and other people. Even though contact may be made with information, knowledge may not be acquired because the information does not comply with current concepts of food or nutrition. If the information seems reasonable, it becomes knowledge and may be implemented to become a part of an individual's food habits.

Sources of nutritional knowledge   The extent of availability of information is surprisingly wide. In the North Central Region of the United States, a sample of middle-income women with preschool children was questioned on where and from whom they had received information on nutrition.[19] A majority of the women (75 per cent) received information during the years they attended school but relatively few women received formal instruction outside the school (twenty-one per cent from youth organizations and two to three per cent from public health or adult education classes).

Persons from whom the mothers obtained information about the food needs of their families included both professional and lay persons (see Table 98).

In addition to personal contact, the mothers reported that they obtained nutrition information from material sources (see Table 99). The results indicate that the mothers were exposed to information on food and nutrition from a variety of sources; the majority of the sources were non-professional in origin.

Table 98   Human sources of nutrition information

	Percentage of sample
Mother or relative	64
Physician	60
Friends or neighbors	29
Home economist, dietitian, nutritionist	22
Dentist	19
Sales persons	6

Source: Fox, H. M., *et al.*, *J. Home Econ.* **62**: 241, 1970.

Table 99   Media sources of nutrition information

	Percentage of sample
Magazines	63
Newpapers	48
Books	47
Television	34
Radio	21
Extension, government bulletins	17
Other sources	3

Source: Fox, H. M., *et al.*, *J. Home Econ.* **62**: 241, 1970.

In a group of young mothers living in Minnesota, the amount of contact with nutrition information in formal classes increased with income level.[5] Approximately 25 per cent remembered attending or participating in group activities where they learned about what foods to eat and how to prepare them. The degree of nutrition knowledge accumulated was associated with the length of formal education and experience in home economics classes. Generally, girls from higher income homes tended to stay in school longer and, in the process, learned more about nutrition than lower-income girls who left school at an earlier age.

Timing of nutrition education   The time of exposure to nutrition education is important. An Israeli study showed the importance of education during childhood.[20] The relative strength of various factors that brought about changes in food habits was determined by asking the source and number of new foods used by a household. A new recipe was considered an indication of influence, whether it was, or was not, nutritionally beneficial. Changes in food habits, increasing from generation to generation, were found in a sample of housewives composed of grandmothers, mothers, and daughters.

The number of new food dishes introduced through the influence of children who had been taught nutrition was evident, indicating the parent's willingness to listen to children and comply with their wishes (see Table 100). There was variation in the degree of adoption within the subgroups of the sample; the rate was higher among Israelis of European origin than Israelis of North African and Near Eastern origin. It is possible the traditional food habits of the European group may have included a wider variety of foods which may have facilitated change.

Table 100   Frequency of introduction of new dishes through various factors

Influencing factor	Per cent of families adoping new dishes	
	Second generation	Third generation
Husband	13	26
Friends or neighbors	40	40
Children	67	91
Food and nutrition meetings	16	55
Newspapers	25	49
Radio	23	35

Source: Bavly, S. J. *Amer. Diet. Assoc.* **48**: 488, 1966.

These studies indicate that there may be an immediate benefit from instructing children in nutrition principles or the effect may not be realized until later, when the children become adult family members. Patterns of accepting new foods or preparing foods in new ways is an important part of nutrition education.

Implementation of nutrition education   An individual must be exposed to information before it can be implemented and used to bring about change. Does the knowledge of the value of a food practice mean that it will be adopted? A group of adult Americans exposed to films on heart disease, cancer, and tuberculosis altered some of their health-related actions but their dietary habits were not markedly changed.[21] A basic requirement for bringing about desirable changes in food habits may be knowledge of how good nutrition status is achieved. Possession of this knowledge, however, is not a guarantee that it will be implemented.

The role of the home and family

Parental attitude   Within the family unit, less tangible psychological factors may also influence food habits. The occurrence of a case of protein calorie malnutrition in a well-educated, middle-class family in the United States demonstrates how poor feeding habits can develop in spite of adequate resources.[22] The infant's febrile reaction to a D. P. T. injection started an acute anxiety on the part of the parents and extreme permissiveness in their attitude towards the diet of the child. Overprotection and overconcern led the parents to adopt a diet of bananas, water, tea, a vitamin preparation and small amounts of meats and cereals blended into the bananas. The diet was fed to the child while he was six to eight months of age and resulted in protein calorie malnutrition.

A permissive attitude, "letting the child eat what he wants", was reported by one-fourth to one-third of the mothers, of a sample of preschool children, in the North Central Region of the United States.[8] The quality of the child's diet suffered when mothers believed the child needed little guidance in food choices. Generally, children who had the lowest total nutrient intake and highest energy intakes had mothers who were most permissive. This suggests that high-calorie diets may be the result of an unrestricted use of "empty calorie" foods. The individuality of the child requires a degree of permissiveness in most areas of behavior, including eating. However, mothers need education that enables them to exercise their permissiveness within a framework insuring an adequate diet.

There was a stong association between personality traits and food choice in a sample of Iowa girls, twelve to fourteen years of age.[23] Girls who chose nutritionally adequate diets possessed more positive personality traits such as emotional stability, conformity, adjustment to reality, and good family relationships than girls with poor diets. As a group, the girls with a highly satisfactory nutrient intake were acquainted with a wider variety of foods than those with a poorer diet. Girls who placed a high value on sociability, independence, status, or enjoyment of food as an end in itself, tended to consider health unimportant, and they were inclined to have an unsatisfactory food intake. When health was considered an important value in selecting food, girls tended to miss fewer meals, to select more adequate meals, and to enjoy food more. Family criticism for not eating the right foods, for eating too much, for eating too often, and for eating too slowly, were associated with the consumption of an inadequate diet.

The relationship between one aspect of the psychological environment of the home and nutritional status of the child was determined in a sample of 150 American children, six to twelve years of age.[24] Children of average weight had higher social adjustment scores, better nutrient intake scores, and parents who had fewer disagreements on child-rearing practices, than overweight or underweight children. The amount of agreement between parents on child-rearing beliefs was strongly related to the nutritional adequacy of the food intake of the child. Deviations from the average body weight, either above or below normal, were related to a lack of agreement between parents. Disagreements between parents on principles of child-rearing may produce an emotional environment conducive to undereating or overeating by the child.

Parents teach food habits consciously, through instruction and by the provision of food, and unconsciously through their own choices and reactions to food served in the household. In addition to this direct influence on the food habits, the young family members are also subject to the influence of the emotional environment of the home. Even though food itself may not be the specific item of contention, general criticism on schoolwork or an atmosphere of disagreement at the family dining table can influence food consumption. In a study of preschool children in the United States, criticism on activity not related to eating, tended to reduce the general level of food consumption and the intake of specific nutrients.[5]

Sociocultural factors and food consumption

An association between sociocultural factors and nutrient intake has been established through the studies referred to in the preceding sections. An adequate diet is clearly related to income and the availability of foods. After determining what foods with high nutrient value are available to a family, other factors come into play to determine the choice of food. The time required to prepare the food and the personal preferences of family members influence choices made in selecting food. Economic restriction, beliefs about food, and a knowledge of nutrient value may all enter the decision-making process, but the interrelationships among these factors are not clear, nor is the order in which they appear.

A model was developed to serve as a framework for a systematic investigation of children's food consumption.[5] This model (see Figure 129) incorporates many of the factors shown in boxes A to M, that are believed to influence food habits.

Motivation and cognition are identified as the main factors influencing food choices, but these two influences are in turn determined by other factors in the environment.

Three factors are associated with "motivation"; these are, first, biological or physiological needs for food related to age, sex, and activity (box A). The second is the psychological need for food and the emotional responses associated with it. The third is the social aspect representing the child's relationships within the family group (box B).

Factors associated with "cognition" include the level of knowledge about food (box C) and the attitudes and values the child holds about specific foods or foods in general (box D).

Two clusters of socioeconomic factors represent variables assumed to influence the development of the "motivation" and "cognition" of the individual. The first cluster, includes the home, the family life cycle state (box E), the social placement, the elements of educational attainment, ethnic group, and religious affiliation (box F), the family's mobility history (box G) and the economic situation (box H). Secondary factors include the knowledge and beliefs about food, the attitudes and values about food, and the time, style and nature of the family's meals. These latter factors are classed as secondary variables because they are affected by the primary socioeconomic factors of the household.

The second cluster of factors influencing the variables of motivation and cognition include the elements related to school. Within the primary group of factors associated with the school there are such elements as the type of school facilities, teaching and administrative staff, class size and the tenor of administration-teacher-parent relationships. Formal nutrition education provided in the classroom and participation in the school lunch program are also assumed to influence the child's food habits (box L), as are the teacher's attitude, knowledge about food and nutrition, and recognition of the importance of nutrition to health (box M).

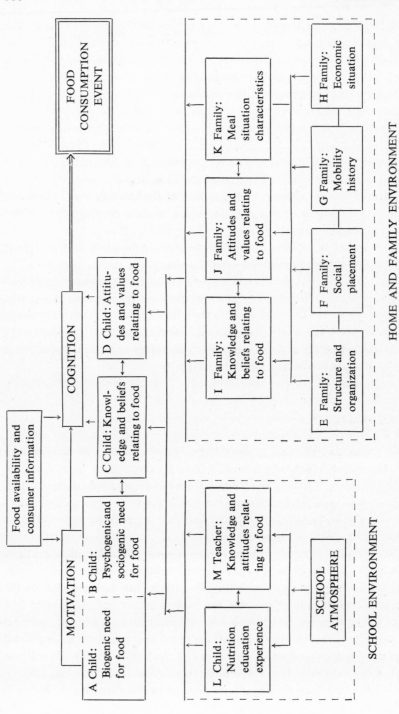

Figure 129   Factors related to a child's food habits (From: Lund, L. Burk, M. *A Multidisciplinary Analysis of Children's Food Consumption Behavior.* Technical Bulletin No. 265. Agricultural Experiment Station, University of Minnesota. 1969)

This model is one suggestion for expressing the interrelationships of the factors which influence food consumption. Similar models could be developed to explain the food habits of an individual, a household, or a community. A schematic analysis prior to attempts to change food habits has considerable advantages. It forces the change agent to identify the determinants of food habits in the problem under consideration. When this has been done, the change agent can decide what factors may be changed. In the case of children, the change agent may decide the school is the only route within the limitation of time and resources. An analysis of the school situation may show that limited student participation in the school lunch program renders it an ineffective means of reaching a majority of students. If there is interest on the part of the teaching staff, the development of a curriculum guide to help teachers integrate nutrition into the classes, may be the method most likely to bring about a change in food habits. This strategy of analysis provides a basis for action and it also brings the situation into perspective for the change agent. It outlines alternatives to which a probability of success can be attached. In any given situation, the odds will be high for success on some factors and low on others. Recognition of the odds against instant success may prepare the change agent for a long term program and prevent the disillusionment which accompanies any project that does not yield immediate results.

Changing food habits

In the history of the human race, shifts and alternations of the diet have occurred without purposeful intervention. Crop failures, pestilence, epidemics, and the devastation caused by wars may alter the pattern of food consumption permanently or temporarily. People migrate as individuals, families or large groups and find different climatic conditions that determine the food supplies. Changes in food patterns occur as human societies borrow from each other, conquer each other, trade and migrate. Urban living dictates new ways of producing and supplying food.

In the midst of all the possibilities for change, families continue to teach children about food. Within the family group, we find the perpetuation of historical patterns which have been developed by a variety of trial-and-error methods in the past. An example of the retention of traditional patterns is found in Israel where spices of the home country are still used with dishes that have been recently adopted.[20]

Channels for communication of information on food are limited to members of the family or the immediate community. Because of these limitations the housewife follows the customs of her mother or grand-mother. Only occasionally are new ways of food preparation introduced by women who join the community. As communications with the outside develop, so do the possibilities increase for acquiring new knowledge about food and nutrition.

During the last half century, the fund of knowledge relating to nutrition has increased enormously but much of this information has not been applied. There is now a trend toward greater use of this information. There are specialists who wish to intervene and to change food habits for the better. It is not essential that there be strict conformity but rather the development of a general pattern of food intake.

Directed change in food habits

When a change in food habits is needed, action may be initiated at two levels. First, the problem may be one best handled through decisions made at the national or state level. These include the enforcement of enrichment, or fortification, of specific food products. Although a child may continue to identify white bread, or polished rice as a high-status food, national or state legislation may enforce the enrichment of the grain with any nutrients that may have been lost through milling. Salt can be fortified with iodine so that the nutrient is supplied even though the food habits of the individual exclude natural sources of iodine.

The second general approach to changing food habits is on the individual or household level. In this case, after the diet is found to be inadequate, an attempt is made to influence the decision-making process of the individual consumer, or the person who is responsible for providing the diet. In addition to employing the usual techniques of persuasion or enticement, efforts are directed toward changing food habits by introducing a new factor, nutrition knowledge.

It is insufficient, however, to provide information in a haphazard or random fashion. There must first be a diagnosis of the prevailing problem and a plan of action. For this latter to be effective, there are two prerequisites to success. First, the foods to be introduced into the diet should be available to the community or households, and second, they should be acceptable, fit into their "way of life" and conform to their customs and attitudes towards food.

The diagnosis of the problem may be facilitated by examining the socio-cultural and economic factors which influence the community, as described earlier in this chapter. There have been many attempts to impart nutritional knowledge in the past, but the effectiveness of educational programs intended to change patterns of food consumption are seldom evaluated in any systematic fashion. Consequently it is difficult to decide why some attempts fail and others succeed. The potential for success should be assessed since an appraisal of difficulties will facilitate the drafting of more realistic plans and time schedules.

The potential for change   Several studies have shown that dietary patterns of households in a community can be compared and ranked according to complexity.[25,26,27] Complex households are distinguished from others in the community by their consumption of a variety of foods in addition to their staple. Households having a relatively complex diet tend to be those that rank high on other measures of complexity. This may be related to educational levels of the adult family members of the household or to the occupation of the household head. Families and households may also be complex with respect to their "way of life" including membership in community groups, contacts with community leaders, and the use of "modern" health practices.

The nutritional problem is seldom an isolated dietetic or food issue. More frequently it is the result of a number of interrelated factors. The complexity should not deter the possibility of change but should arouse caution in proposing change. The recognition of the complexity of the causation provides a more realistic view of the possibility of change.

Most people will accept that food habits are intimately bound to many aspects of life, yet they will reject the idea that a change in food habits may be impossible within the existing conditions of a household or community. Even where habits are rigidly controlled an expert would probably be able to suggest a workable method of improving the diet. Many specialists do not appreciate that the consumer may not be able to accept the suggestion. For example, a mother of six children may feed her family a limited diet consisting mainly of rice. She may be offered sound advice on how to improve the family diet. She declines the offer because she cannot afford the risk of changing to a new system. She knows that survival is possible on her present food pattern and intake, but the narrow economic margin on which she operates does not allow her to adopt another system with its attendant risks. People may be unable to say why they refuse to accept sound nutritional advice, but this does not mean they have no reason for refusal, or they have not understood the message conveyed by the specialist.

There is no infallible method for predicting the extent of change which may be expected in the food habits of groups or individuals. One index may be the degree of complexity that is exhibited in other aspects of life. There is reason to believe that change may be more likely to take place in families who have achieved more education, more contacts outside the community, or who may be more involved with community affairs. Families such as these may have relatively less need than others, but they may be in an economic, social, and psychological position to use proferred advice. The expert might well be advised to identify such households as a target for education. The specialist who bases a choice on the potential for change, plus need, has a greater probability of success than the specialist who directs advice on the basis of need alone.

One indication of the potential of the family for change may be the degree of innovativeness in the existing food habits. Collecting and using new recipes indicates a willingness to try new ideas and an interest in preparing food in different ways.

If there is no obvious way to assess the potential for change, the educator may test for this. Working with the household or individual on a specific problem presents opportunities to observe ways to improve the dietary pattern. However, it may only be possible to promote one small change at a time. This technique lends itself to application in situations similar to that previously described where a mother feeds her children mainly on rice. The addition of an inexpensive but nutritious item to the diet might be a financial risk she would accept although a general reorganization of the basic diet would be refused. For example, she may be willing to include beans in the diet; these are inexpensive but the protein acts as an excellent supplement to rice protein. The change is justified on a nutritional basis and would cost very little. If one suggestion can be implemented, then others may be followed.

When a family appears to have no prospects of innovation because of economic limitations, ignorance, or beliefs, there may be very little opportunity for change no matter how necessary it seems. Such hopeless situations are unfortunately prevalent in impoverished countries and it seems that the greatest chance for improvement lies in the provision of temporary relief. This may be material or financial; without such help, prospects of improvement are minimal. The risk of perpetuating a continuous welfare service for such populations may have to be carefully studied.

Role of the educator   There are two primary elements that are essential to the success of any educational venture.[28] The first is the possession of appropriate knowledge and skills and the second is a detailed understanding of the economic, social, and cultural conditions of the target community.

These conclusions were reached by social antropologists who studied programs intended to improve standards of nutritional health. The failure of cookery classes held in a health center was attributable to these two criteria being ignored. The classes proved to be more popular with the well-to-do women than with the mothers of families most in need of nutritional improvement. The setting and utensils used in the demonstrations had little resemblance to those found in the poorer homes and the poorer women could not have put the instruction into practice. Before there can be any change in food habits, learning must occur within the mind of the recipient who must recognize the possibilities for implementing the new knowledge.

The achievement of change depends upon the change agent, the choice of the specific advice to be offered, and its method of presentation. Presenting material by lecture, or by "telling", is a traditional method of instruction and assumes that if the recipient knows the value of a practice, then the practice will be followed. It is important to realize, however, that hearing implies more than being within voice range. Learning occurs only when a new concept is received by the senses and is placed into the background of knowledge already held by the individual. Persuading a mother to include vitamin C rich fruits and vegetables in the meals she serves her family entails beginning at her level of understanding of the need for these foods. The fact that citrus fruits contain vitamin C which prevents scurvy may not impress a mother with a limited understanding of nutrition and who has never seen scurvy. Her concept of food may include a relationship between food and growth or perhaps a simpler idea of the need for food. Every person has their own mental image of food. At the basic level it is a substance that prevents hunger. To expand this idea until it eventually encompasses what the specialist has in mind, may require many preliminary steps. The specialist who operates from a fairly highly developed concept may be speaking the same language but the mental images in the mind of the specialist and the recipient may bear no resemblance to each other. To learn something new, the individual must be assisted in enlarging his existing views. An educator can teach but this is of no value unless there is learning by the recipient. To increase the possibility of learning, the method of teaching and the material used must be carefully adjusted to the capabilities of the learner.

The principle of emphasizing the improvement of a current dietary pattern rather than change should be employed when working with individuals and families. This approach is positive and avoids the implication of error.

An atmosphere free of condemnation is essential if a good working relationship is to be established. To demonstrate an understanding of the situation, the suggestions offered must be ones that can be attained by the household and can be justified by reasons within the comprehension of the housewife.

Techniques for implementing Change

Opinion leaders The shotgun approach of attempting to reach as many women as possible in a community is often used by the specialist. This is because of the poor tools that are available for selecting a more effective distribution system for the information. Conveying the same information to everyone violates the principle of beginning instruction on the learner's level of understanding. In any group there will be varying degrees of background information and the instructor may structure the material in too elementary a fashion for some and too complex a form for others. By working with a small group of women who are assumed to be the local leaders, the specialist has an opportunity to determine the level of information held by the participants.

Opinion leaders are persons who are assumed to affect the behavior or attitudes of those with whom they come into contact. However, the women who are leaders in other areas of community life may not be those who are influental in determining food habits. An important aspect of opinion leadership is that leadership is not general; opinion leaders are usually leaders in one area.[29]

Ideally, the most effective way of spreading nutrition information through a community would be to work with the women who are already designated as the opinion leaders in food and nutrition. Assiduous searching may be the only way of locating them. Very little is known about identifying food opinion leaders and there is no method of easy identification. A food opinion leader may be the woman who is acknowledged to be the best cook in the neighborhood, one whose recipes are highly prized, or one who is known to "set a good table" for her family.

A nutrition education program based on friendship groups has been attempted in a low-income area in the United States.[30] Potential leaders were first picked among the women known to local health workers as leaders in community life. These women were asked to invite five or six friends to a "nutrition luncheon" as guests of the leaders. The purpose of the luncheon was to interest the women in nutrition and encourage the formation of a group that would continue to meet and, with the assistance of the nutritionist, learn more about nutrition. Few of the community leaders agreed to cooperate and those that did so failed to continue beyond the initial luncheon. The natural friendship group pattern was not an effective method for diffusing information on nutrition; the introduction of an ulterior motive seemed to render this pattern ineffective. In most communities there already exist strong local groups that could be effective in spreading nutrition information. The group might be a social club, business club, a church group or one of the more informal groups formed in villages at the market place or clothes washing site.

The target of nutrition education has usually been the female household head. There is basis for this choice. If food moves through a stepwise progression; purchase, storage, preparation, and serving, the person who should be influenced is the gatekeeper who moves the food through the channels.[3] The woman of the household is often the primary gatekeeper, although the male household head often does the shopping in many societies. In households where the male purchases the food supplies and a servant does the preparation and serving, instructing the female may be an academic exercise that has little effect on changing the food habits of the household.

The male houshold head may exert an influence on the food consumption patterns of the household in a less direct way than purchasing food. In a study of a Ghanaian community, it was found that the education, level of literacy, nutrition knowledge, and number of information sources of the woman were related to the pattern of foods served in the home.[26] However, if the female had a higher level of education, literacy, and other characteristics than the male, the potential benefit upon household practices, including dietary pattern, was not realized. If this is true in other households, educating the woman beyond the level achieved by the male household head may yield negligible results in terms of changing household practices. Even though the evidence is slight, it does indicate that nutrition education should not be aimed solely at women.

Attitude change Learning theorists using the principle of reinforcement would predict that the most effective way to change attitudes would be to stimulate a change in behavior related to the new attitude and then to re-inforce that behavior. The practical problem is that often there is no method available for eliciting the desired behavior. Nevertheless, the matter is one of interest, and psychologists have attempted to design experiments to test this theory of attitude change.

One study designed to test for attitude change was based on the following hypothesis: If a person can be induced to do or say something which is

18*

contrary to his private opinion, there will be a tendency for him to change his opinion so as to bring it into correspondence with what he has said or done. However, the greater the pressure employed to bring about the overt behavior, the weaker will be the tendency to change opinions.[31] A group of subjects were exposed to a set of boring tasks and then paid to tell a second group that their experience had been enjoyable and interesting. When the first group received a reasonable award, their expression of enjoyment of the task increased. When, however, the reward was high their change in attitude was relatively small.

A similar attempt was made to change attitudes within the context of changing food habits. During World War II, Levin organized informal groups of women to discuss methods of improving diets.[3] Lectures by nutritionists were less effective in incorporating specific meat items into the diet than the discussion methods where the specialist was present as a resource person. Individuals who participated in discussions leading to a decision, subsequently included the food items more often than individuals who were told the value of specific food habits. When there was a public commitment voicing an affirmative opinion during the meeting, it was more likely that the practice would be applied in the individual's own home.

The tendency to follow a practice if it is personally advocated was found in an educational project in Mississippi.[31] Program aides were trained to instruct clients in the use of commodity foods and food stamps provided by the Federal government. Four "lessons" were taught. Program aides, who were also welfare clients, showed significantly more improvement in their food habits than the women who received instruction in their homes or those who received instruction during visits to the food distribution centers. The aides were taught by professional home economists and this factor may have influenced the outcome but it seems likely that their behavior was influenced by supporting the practice in public.

Selecting recipients for nutrition education on the basis of their roles as community leaders seems to be a useful technique for disseminating information. The level of instruction can be adjusted to their initial level of understanding of nutrition and they are in a position to act as instructors to other women in the community. If they do agree to undertake the task of teaching nutrition principles to other women, it is likely there will be a tendency for them to adopt the practices they recommend.

Nutrition education of children   For many years the importance of instructing children in nutrition has been advocated in the belief that the pattern of later life may be affected by influencing food habits during the years they are developing. Education in nutrition may be achieved by formal instruction or more informally by participation in school meals.

Not many people would disagree with the value of nutrition education for children. However, the level of motivation for learning about food and nutrition may be higher later in life when the children are grown and establishing their own homes. One difficulty has been in developing an effective course of study within the school curriculum. Nutrition need not be taught as an isolated unit but can be incorporated into such subjects as reading and social studies at the elementary level. This requires a curriculum guide with suggestions for the conceptual development of the subject matter. The traditional method of teaching the value of food by the "Basic Four" food groups: meat, milk, vegetables, and cereals, need not be retaught at every level. This model for guiding food choices is merely one level of developing the concept of selecting an adequate diet.

The New York State program in the health sciences has several innovative aspects.[32] The underlying philosophy is that the study of health affairs must be based upon an understanding of human ecology, the study of man in interaction with his environment. The content areas in the health sciences course of study are illustrated in Figure 130.

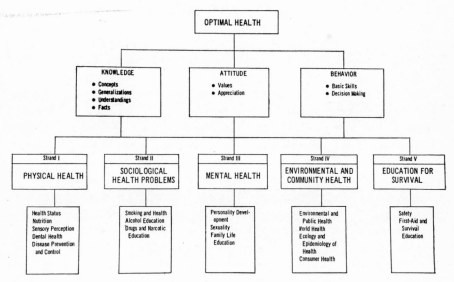

Figure 130   Content and Basic Aims of New York Education Program. (Reproduced from Prototype Curriculum Materials for the Elementary and Secondary Grades — Strand 1. Physical Health. With the permission of Dr. John Sinacore and acknowledgment to the New York State Education Department, Albany, New York).

The syllabus for each course offered in the program follows a four-column format. The first column is a reference outline of the material covered. The second column lists the major understandings and fundamental concepts to be learned by the student. The third column includes suggested teaching aids and learning activities. The last column consists of supplementary information for the teacher. For example, the first page of the syllabus for the primary grades is divided as follows:[33]

References	Major Understandings and Fundamental Concepts	Suggested Teaching Aids and Learning Activities	Supplementary Information for the Teacher
What is food?	A. All living things need food and water —Plants get their food from water, sunlight, air, and soil	(1) Grow plants from seeds with and without fertilizer	A lima bean produces a rapidly growing plant

Nutrition is one of the courses of study within Strand 1, Physical Health. The major understandings and fundamental concepts to be included at the various grade levels of the nutrition section are as follows:

Strand 1. Physical Health. Nutrition for Kindergarten to Grade 3

The curriculum is directed toward developing positive attitudes to food, accepting a variety of foods, appreciating eating as a pleasurable experience, realizing that people eat in many different ways, and beginning to understand the relation of food to health and growth. Much can be integrated with other subjects: social studies, arithmetic, spelling, reading, and art. It is important to realize at this level that activities which help children act in a desired way are more effective than talking about the desired behavior.

Strand 1. Physical Health. Nutrition for Grades 4, 5, and 6

The nutrition curriculum for the intermediate grades is directed toward helping the student to discover in some detail how food is related to health and growth and to understand the role of criteria for selecting food. It also provides an opportunity for the student to develop a concept of the food people eat as an integral part of the physical and sociocultural environment.

Strand 1. Physical Health. Nutrition for Grades 7. 8, and 9

The nutrition curriculum at this level is directed toward helping the student explore in more detail the relationships among nutrition, health, disease, heredity and environment, and providing the opportunity for him to apply his knowledge of nutrition to practical situations. The rapid changes which the adolescent undergoes physically and psychologically focus his attention on the practical problems he encounters. Nutrition teaching should provide opportunity for the student to analyze his own practices in the persepctive of sound background knowledge.

Strand 1. Physical Health. Nutrition for Grades 10, 11, and 12

The curriculum seeks to take advantage of the highschool student's keen interest in, and awareness of, events in the society and world around him, and in his own future. Units on nutrition problems in developing countries, hunger in the United States, and obesity in an affluent society seek to help the student relate his nutrition knowledge to his concern for others. Units on prenatal and infant nutrition and the responsibility of the individual and the community for nutrition pose questions and problems that are significant to the student as he approaches adult independence.

The curriculum developed by the University of New York is an example of a graded sequence of material which introduces basic concepts of nutrition and subsequently enlarges and adds to the basic concepts. A program of in-service training for teachers accompanies the introduction of the syllabus for each course into the curriculum.

There has been a great deal written about the value of school meals as a means for improving nutritional status and as a method of teaching good food habits. It can be demonstrated that the food intake of children from homes with inadequate resources is improved by participation in school lunch programs in the United States.[34]

The educational value of the program is not clear. Even when there are no alternatives to the school cafeteria, such as vending machines, restaurants, or packed lunches, children still have the option to refuse unfamiliar foods included in the menu for educational purposes. If lunches are provided as a service that is to be well-used the meals tend to be adjusted to the preferences of the children. Complaints from students and teachers are all too common in a school cafeteria. Perhaps part of the difficulty lies in the fact that the cafeteria is usually a service with no responsibility residing with students or teachers. Conveying criticism or suggestions to the cafeteria staff does not constitute sharing the responsibility for its

operation. To make a school lunch program a part of the school curriculum requires planning and commitment by the teachers. Class projects
including menu planning should elicit some feeling of responsibility among
students in addition to supplementing classroom teaching. The key to the
effectiveness of a school lunch program as a teaching tool lies in making
the program a shared responsibility rather than merely a service or place
to keep the children during the noon hour.

In the introduction to this book it was emphasized that the various
sciences and disciplines in nutrition have pursued their own interests.
An enormous wealth of knowledge has been accumulated. Mostly it related
to nutrition problems and only a small part is applied to their solution.
Many of the suggestions for improved nutritional status are based on sound
theoretical considerations. However, so little is known of the difficulties
that are involved in bringing about change that the impracticability of the
suggestions remains generally unrecognized.

For example, it has been suggested that the protein deficiency diseases
of Asia and Africa can be prevented by producing more protein-rich foods.
The problems of distributing and marketing these foods in areas where
they are really required is very often unrecognized. It is also not realized
that if the communities had an efficient distributing and marketing system
they would probably not be suffering from protein deficiency disease.

There are signs that nutrition is being recognized now as a subject of
great breadth. This is an important fact that has been obscured for the last
thirty to forty years, by the search for knowledge in depth. Because nutrition
is a broad subject it should not be assumed to be lacking in depth. No one
discipline can be responsible for nutrition, each is complementary to the
other. It should be accepted that the behavioral scientist is as important
a member of the nutrition team as the biochemist, and that the role of
community nutritionist is as significant as that of the food technologist.
The knowledge and skills of the one can not be applied successfully without
the knowledge, skills and collaboration of the other. It is hoped that this
text may have helped the student to appreciate the broad implications of
nutrition and to see where their respective interests and abilities may be
used to help bring about a global improvement in nutritional status.

References

1. Adelson, S. F. "Changes in Diets of Households, 1955–1965." *J. Home Econ.* **60**: 448,
   1968
2. Mead, M. Culture Change in Relation to Nutrition, p. 51. In *Malnutrition and Food
   Habits*. Eds. Burgess,A., Dean, R.F.A. New York: 1962.

3. Lewin, K. Forces Behind Food Habits and Methods of Change. In *The Problem of Changing Food Habits.* Bulletin No. 108, p. 35. Report of the Committee on Food Habits. National Research Council, Washington, D.C. 1943.

4. Eppright, E. S., Fox, H. M., Fryer, B. A., Lamkin, G. H., Vivian, V. M. "Eating Behavior of Preschool Children." *J. Nutr. Educ.* **1**: 16, Summer 1969.

5. Lund, L. A., Burk, M. C. A Multidisciplinary Analysis of Children's Food Consumption Behavior. Technical Bulletin No. 265. Agricultural Experiment Station, University of Minnesota, 1969.

6. Dube, S. C. *Indian Village.* London: Routledge and Kegan, Paul, 1955.

7. Latham, M. C., Robson, J. R. K. "A Trial to Evaluate the Benefit of Different Protein Rich Foods to African School Children." *Nutr. Dieta* **7**: 28, 1965

8. Eppright, E. S., Fox, H. M., Fryer, B. A., Lamkin, G. H., Vivian, V. M. "Nutrition Knowledge and Attitudes of Mothers." *J. Home Econ.* **62**: 327, 1970.

9. Captain, O. B., McIntire, M. S. "Cost and Quality of Food in Poverty and Non-Poverty Urban Areas." *J. Amer. Dietet. Ass.* **55**: 569, 1969.

10. Meyers, T. "The Extra Cost of Being Poor." *J. Home Econ.* **62**: 379, 1970.

11. Harris, P. T. Effects of Foods and Nutrition Education on Food Practices of Low Income Families in Four Mississippi Counties, Summer 1966. Home Economics Series No. 3. Mississippi State University, Agricultural Experiment Station, 1967.

12. Bivens, G. E. "Convenience Foods 1955 and 1965." *J. Home Econ.* **61**: 26, 1969.

13. Jerome, N. W. "Northern Urbanization and Food Consumption Patterns of Southern-Born Negroes." *Amer. J. Clin. Nutr.* **22**: 1667, 1969.

14. Pyke, M. "Scientific Technology and the Mercenary Society." *J. Nutr. Educ.* **1**: 20, Winter 1970.

15. Devadas, R. P. "Social and Cultural Factors Influencing Malnutrition." *J. Home Econ.* **62**: 164, 1970.

16. Mazess, R. B. "Home-Cold Food Beliefs Among Andean Peasants." *J. Amer. Dietet. Ass.* **53**: 109, 1968.

17. Nyoiti, S. *Macrobiotics—The Astonishing Oriental Plan for Total Health.* New York: Award Books, 1970.

18. Sherlock, P., Rothchild, E. O. "Scurvy Produced by a Zen Macrobiotic Diet." *J. Amer. Med. Ass.* **199**: 794, 1967.

19. Fox, H. M., Fryer, B. A., Lamkin, G. H., Vivian, V. M., Eppright, E. S. "The North Central Regional Study of Diets of Preschool Children. 1. Family Environment." *J. Home Econ.* **62**: 241, 1970.

20. Bavly, S. "Changes in Food Habits in Israel." *J. Amer. Dietet. Ass.* **48**: 488, 1966.

21. Haefner, D. P., Kirscht, J. P. "Motivational and Behavioral Effects of Modifying Health Beliefs." *Pub. Hlth. Rep.* **85**: 478, 1970.

22. Shappley, B. G., Williams, T. E., Birdsong, M. Donaldson, M. H. "Kwashiorkor with Psychologic Etiology." *Clin Ped.* **8**: 709, 1969.

23. Hinton, M. A., Eppright, E. S., Chadderdon, H., Wolins, L. "Eating Behavior and Dietary Intake of Girls 12 to 14 Years Old." *J. Amer. Dietet. Ass.* **43**: 223, 1963.

24. Wakefield, L. M., Merrow, S. B. "Interrelationships Between Selected Nutritional, Clinical, and Sociological Measurements of Preadolescent Children From Independent Low Income Families." *Amer. J. Clin. Nutr.* **20**: 291, 1967.

25. Sanjur, D., Cravioto, J., Rosales, L., Van Veen, A. "Infant Feeding and Weaning Practices in a Rural Preindustrial Setting." *Acta Paed. Scand.* Supplement 200, 1970.

26. Larkin, F. A., Owen, C., Rhodes, K. "Differentiation of Households in a Ghanaian Community." *J. Marriage and the Family* **32**: 304, 1970.
27. Chassey, J., Van Veen, A., Young, F. W. "The Application of Social Science Research Methods to the Study of Food Habits and Food Consumption in an Industrializing Area." *Amer. J. Clin. Nutr.* **20**: 56, 1967.
28. Burgess, A. "Nutrition Education in Public Health Programs—What Have We Learned?" *Amer. J. Public Health* **51**: 1715, 1961.
29. Katz, E., Lazarsfeld, P. *Personal Influence.* The Free Press, 1964.
30. Koos, E. L. A Study of the Use of the Friendship Pattern in Nutrition Education. In *The Problem of Changing Food Habits.* Bulletin No. 108. Report of the Committee on Food Habits. National Research Council. Washington, D.C. 1943.
31. Festinger, L., Carlsmith, J. M. "Cognitive Consequences of Forced Compliance." *J. Abnormal and Soc. Psychol.* **58**: 203, 1959.
32. Sinacore, J. S. "New York State's Program in the Health Sciences." *The Bulletin of the National Association of Secondary-School Principals.* **52**: 81, 1969.
33. Prototype Curriculum Materials for the Elementary and Secondary Grades—Strand 1. Physical Health. Nutrition for Grades K-3. Grades 4–6, Grades 7–9, and Grades 10–12. The University of the State of New York. The State Education Department, Bureau of Secondary Curriculum Development, Albany, New York 1970.
34. Larkin, F. A., Sandretto, A. M. "Dietary Patterns and the Use of Commodity Foods in a Potawotami Indian Community." *J. Home Econ.* **62**: 385, 1970

Index

595

19*